Ruminant Ophthalmology

Editor

ANNETTE M. O'CONNOR

VETERINARY CLINICS
OF NORTH AMERICA:
FOOD ANIMAL PRACTICE

www.vetfood.theclinics.com

Consulting Editor
ROBERT A. SMITH

July 2021 • Volume 37 • Number 2

ELSEVIER

1600 John F. Kennedy Boulevard • Suite 1800 • Philadelphia, Pennsylvania, 19103-2899

http://www.vetfood.theclinics.com

VETERINARY CLINICS OF NORTH AMERICA: FOOD ANIMAL PRACTICE Volume 37, Number 2
July 2021 ISSN 0749-0720, ISBN-13: 978-0-323-81315-0

Editor: Katerina Heidhausen
Developmental Editor: Axell Ivan Jade M. Purificacion

Veterinary Clinics of North America: Food Animal Practice (ISSN 0749-0720) is published in March, July, and November by Elsevier Inc., 360 Park Avenue South, New York, NY 10010-1710. Subscription prices are $262.00 per year (domestic individuals), $628.00 per year (domestic institutions), $100.00 per year (domestic students/residents), $283.00 per year (Canadian individuals), $672.00 per year (Canadian institutions), $335.00 per year (international individuals), $672.00 per year (international institutions), $100.00 per year (Canadian students), and $165.00 (international students). To receive student/resident rate, orders must be accompanied by name of affiliated institution, date of term, and the signature of program/residency coordinator on institution letterhead. *Clinics* subscription prices. All prices are subject to change without notice. **POSTMASTER:** Send address changes to *Veterinary Clinics of North America: Food Animal Practice*, Elsevier Health Sciences Division, Subscription Customer Service, 3251 Riverport Lane, Maryland Heights, MO 63043. Customer Service (orders, claims, online, change of address): Elsevier Health Sciences Division, Subscription **Customer Service, 3251 Riverport Lane, Maryland Heights, MO 63043. Tel: 1-800-654-2452 (U.S. and Canada); 314-447-8871 (ouside U.S. and Canada). Fax: 314-447-8029. E-mail: journalscustomerservice-usa@elsevier.com (for print support); journalsonlinesupport-usa@elsevier.com (for online support).**

Reprints. For copies of 100 or more, of articles in this publication, please contact the Commercial Reprints Department, Elsevier Inc., 360 Park Avenue South, New York, NY 10010-1710. Tel.: 212-633-3874; Fax: 212-633-3820; E-mail: reprints@elsevier.com.

Veterinary Clinics of North America: Food Animal Practice is covered in *Current Contents/Agriculture, Biology and Environmental Sciences, MEDLINE/PubMed (Index Medicus), and Excerpta Medica.*

Printed in the United States of America.

Contributors

CONSULTING EDITOR

ROBERT A. SMITH, DVM, MS
Diplomate, American Board of Veterinary Practitioners; Veterinary Research and Consulting Services, LLC, Greeley, Colorado, USA; Veterinary Research and Consulting Services, LLC, Stillwater, Oklahoma, USA

EDITOR

ANNETTE M. O'CONNOR, BVSc, MVSc, DVSc, FANZCVS
Professor of Epidemiology and Chairperson, Department of Large Animal Clinical Sciences, College of Veterinary Medicine, Michigan State University, East Lansing, Michigan, USA

AUTHORS

JOHN A. ANGELOS, DVM, PhD
Diplomate, American College of Veterinary Internal Medicine; Professor, Department of Medicine and Epidemiology, School of Veterinary Medicine, University of California, Davis, California, USA

MICHAEL L. CLAWSON, PhD
Research Molecular Biologist, U.S. Meat Animal Research Center, USDA Agriculture Research Service, Nebraska, USA

KRISTIN A. CLOTHIER, DVM, PhD
Diplomate, American College of Veterinary Microbiologists; Department of Pathology, Microbiology, and Immunology, Associate Professor and Veterinary Microbiologist, California Animal Health and Food Safety Laboratory System, School of Veterinary Medicine, University of California, Davis, Davis, California, USA

ELLIOTT J. DENNIS, PhD
Department of Agricultural Economics, University of Nebraska-Lincoln, Lincoln, Nebraska, USA

BINH DOAN, BS
Carver College of Medicine, University of Iowa, Iowa City, Iowa, USA

PAOLA ELIZALDE, DVM, MS
PhD Candidate, School of Public Health, University of Saskatchewan, Saskatoon, Saskatchewan, Canada

PHILIP GRIEBEL, DVM, PhD
Professor, School of Public Health, Research Scientist, VIDO-Intervac, University of Saskatchewan, Saskatoon, Saskatchewan, Canada

MATTHEW HILLE, DVM
Veterinary Resident, Nebraska Veterinary Diagnostic Center, School of Veterinary Medicine and Biomedical Sciences, University of Nebraska-Lincoln, Lincoln, Nebraska, USA

MAC KNEIPP, BVSc, MVS, MANZCVS
Veterinary Clinician, Sydney School of Veterinary Science, The University of Sydney, Camden, New South Wales, Australia

JOHN DUSTIN LOY, DVM, PhD
Diplomate, American College of Veterinary Microbiologists; Associate Professor and Veterinary Microbiologist, Nebraska Veterinary Diagnostic Center, School of Veterinary Medicine and Biomedical Sciences, University of Nebraska-Lincoln, Lincoln, Nebraska, USA

GABRIELE MAIER, DVM, MPVM, PhD
Diplomate, American College of Veterinary Preventive Medicine; Assistant Specialist in Cooperative Extension, Department of Population Health and Reproduction, School of Veterinary Medicine, University of California, Davis, Davis, California, USA

ANNETTE M. O'CONNOR, BVSc, MVSc, DVSc, FANZCVS
Professor of Epidemiology and Chairperson, Department of Large Animal Clinical Sciences, College of Veterinary Medicine, Michigan State University, East Lansing, Michigan, USA

DAVID SHEEDY, DVM, MPVM
Veterinary Medicine Teaching and Research Center, School of Veterinary Medicine, University of California, Davis, Tulare, California, USA

Contents

Pinkeye and infectious bovine keratoconjunctivitis (IBK) are imprecise terms that describe diverse ocular diseases. Moraxella bovis is the major causative agent of IBK; however, disease epidemiology is not fully known. Not all cases referred to as pinkeye are of infectious origin, and not all IBK involve M bovis. This article suggests the term pinkeye should no longer be used, offers a case definition for IBK (a herd disease), and suggests describing ocular signs of IBK using existing clinical descriptors rather than resorting to novel scores. A new term "ocular moraxellosis" is defined as IBK from which Moraxella spp are demonstrated.

Studies have sought to develop effective vaccines against infectious bovine keratoconjunctivitis (IBK). Most research has focused on parenterally administered vaccines against *Moraxella bovis* antigens; however, researchers have also included *Moraxella bovoculi* antigens in vaccines to prevent IBK. Critical knowledge gaps remain as to which *Moraxella* spp antigens might be completely protective, and whether systemic, mucosal, or both types of immune responses are required for protection against IBK associated with *Moraxella* spp. Immune responses to commensal *Moraxella* spp residing in the upper respiratory tract and eye have not been analyzed to determine if these responses control colonization or contribute to IBK.

Establishing causation, otherwise known as causal assessment, is a difficult task, made more difficult by the variety of causal assessment frameworks available to consider. In this article, Bradford Hill viewpoints are used to discuss the evidence base for Moraxella bovis and Moraxella bovoculi being component causes of infectious bovine keratoconjunctivitis. Each of the nine Bradford Hill viewpoints are introduced and explained: strength, consistency, specificity, temporality, biologic gradient, plausibility, coherence, experiment, and analogy. Examples of how the viewpoints have been applied for other causal relations are provided, and then the evidence base for M bovis and M bovoculi is discussed.

less than 0.15, except for some estimates for Herefords and Angus cattle around 0.2 and 1 study reporting a heritability of 0.33. These magnitudes of heritability are typically described as low to moderate. Quantitative trait locus on chromosome 1, 2, 12, 13, 20, and 21 has been associated with IBK resistance.

In this article, the evidence base for treating infectious bovine kera-toconjunctivitis (IBK) is discussed. First, we summarize the available evidence for antibiotic treatments registered in North America. We then discuss the evidence base for nonantibiotic alternatives. We do not discuss antibiotic treatments that do not use registered protocols; such information is available in another review. Finally, we discuss how the research community could generate more evidence for effective treatments and the comparative efficacy information to help veterinarians and producers decide between treatment options.

Pili and cytotoxins are important virulence factors and antigens for Morax-ella spp. Local and systemic immunity may play a role in the body's response to infectious bovine keratoconjunctivitis (IBK). No evidence exists that eliminating the carrier state for IBK is possible or beneficial. Evidence for efficacious transfer of passive immunity from dams to calves is conflicting. Autogenous vaccines and commercial vaccines for putative pathogens for IBK have not yet shown efficacy in blinded randomized field trials. Study design features, such as randomization, blinding, diagnostic criteria, and use of a placebo, reduce the risk of bias in vaccine studies for IBK.

A summary of available literature on the prevalence and estimated economic impacts of infectious bovine keratoconjunctivitis (IBK) from around the world is made. Country-level prevalence of IBK has been reported only for the United States, Australia, and New Zealand. We provide an estimate of IBK prevalence rate by geographic climate and region accounting for cattle sub-species and age. Estimated prevalence worldwide is 2.78%. Historical economic impact assessments are available only for the United States, Australia, and United Kingdom. Rarely do assessments capture the full economic cost of the disease. Better data on prevalence and how treatment and prevention decisions modify disease impacts is required to estimate the global economic impact.

In this article, the authors summarize the future needs from a research perspective to make the greatest gains. They discuss the areas of research: diagnosis, epidemiology, economic impact, prevention, and treatment. In some areas, simple studies with little cost could be conducted that would quickly add to the evidence base. In other areas, substantial investment is needed if new study approaches, which do not repeat past studies' failures, are to be conducted. To maximize the value of research funding, it is essential to critically evaluate the information gains from prior studies and ensure that studies increase knowledge incrementally.

VETERINARY CLINICS OF NORTH AMERICA: FOOD ANIMAL PRACTICE

SERIES OF RELATED INTEREST

Veterinary Clinics: Equine Practice
https://www.vetequine.theclinics.com/

THE CLINICS ARE NOW AVAILABLE ONLINE!
Access your subscription at:
www.theclinics.com

Preface

Infectious Bovine Keratoconjunctivitis

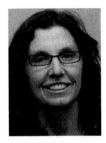

Annette M. O'Connor, BVSc, MVSc, DVSc, FANZCVS
Editor

In this issue of the *Veterinary Clinics of North America: Food Animal Practice*, we focus on infectious bovine keratoconjunctivitis (IBK). I want to begin by thanking all the authors who contributed to this particular issue. When they agreed to write for this special issue, they did not know about the severe acute respiratory syndrome coronavirus 2 pandemic and its impact on their workload. While trying to provide service to clients and maintain research laboratories, and the ever-changing expectations for teaching during 2020 and 2021, they were gracious and patient as we put this special issue together.

IBK is the most important ocular disease of cattle because of its impact on animal health, animal well-being, the antibiotic usage treatment required, and its effect on production. IBK has been the subject of research for over 60 years. When I was in veterinary school, I was told that IBK was caused by *Moraxella bovis*. I took this knowledge to be a known fact and was under the impression for many years that IBK was a simple disease caused by a singular organism. The evidence that *M bovis* is causal is available; however, that does not mean that IBK is the simple disease I had been taught as a veterinary student. In reading this special issue, it will become evident that many questions remain about all the factors that contribute to the development of IBK. What causes some herds to have consistently high levels of IBK and others to have low or no IBK is still not understood. Furthermore, we do not understand why within a herd, some animals develop IBK and others do not.

Although I have said much is unknown, that does not mean progress is not being made. We are in a much better place in our knowledge of IBK than we were 10 years ago, and so it is important to summarize the state of knowledge about IBK. In this issue, the articles focus on different aspects of IBK. The issue begins with a discussion about the diagnosis at the individual and herd level. The next article discusses the all-important immunology of the eye, a critical factor for understanding how we might

Vet Clin Food Anim 37 (2021) xi–xii
https://doi.org/10.1016/j.cvfa.2021.04.001
0749-0720/21/© 2021 Published by Elsevier Inc.

vetfood.theclinics.com

prevent IBK. This immunology article is followed by an article on establishing causation and applying those concepts to IBK. If we are seeking to understand what causes IBK, we must know how we reach causal inference. The articles on the disease's epidemiology focus on the epidemiological triad of pathogen, environment, and host. The next articles of the issue discuss the prevention of IBK, the treatment of IBK, and understanding the economic impact of IBK. The final article about where we can go as a research community highlights the importance of continued research on this topic. There has been a resurgence of research about IBK, particularly in vaccines and molecular approaches to disease epidemiology, in recent years. This resurgence is leading to really interesting findings that will help us understand the disease better and create more options for designing effective control programs.

Annette M. O'Connor, BVSc, MVSc, DVSc, FANZCVS
Department of Large Animal
Clinical Sciences
College of Veterinary Medicine
Michigan State University
784 Wilson Road, Room G-100
East Lansing, MI 48824, USA

E-mail address:
oconn445@msu.edu

Defining and Diagnosing Infectious Bovine Keratoconjunctivitis

Mac Kneipp, BVSc, MVS, MANZCVS

KEYWORDS

- Cattle • Infectious bovine keratoconjunctivitis • Pinkeye • Moraxellosis
- Case definition • Diagnosis

KEY POINTS

- Pinkeye and infectious bovine keratoconjunctivitis (IBK) are imprecise terms.
- There is no case definition for IBK.
- To diagnose IBK there are no pathognomonic clinical signs.
- IBK is a herd disease.

INTRODUCTION

For more than 130 years, there have been reports from around the world of a contagious disease confined to the eyes of cattle, variously called keratitis contagiosa, infectious keratitis, contagious ophthalmia, New Forest eye, blight, pinkeye, and infectious bovine keratoconjunctivitis (IBK). In 1889, Billings[1] described "keratitis contagiosa" in Nebraska dairy cows, "by no means a new disease." In 1897, Penberthy[2] reported on 4 outbreaks in England of "contagious ophthalmia." In 1911, Poels,[3] in Holland, reported on "keratitis infectiosa," a disease known for many years in many countries.

Despite becoming a well-recognized herd syndrome with acute onset, there is no case definition; that is, criteria to decide if an animal or herd has the disease or not. Lack of case definition is a possible source of misclassification bias[4] and complicates diagnosis, treatment, and prevention.[5] Disease terminology and definitions vary among cattle producers, veterinarians, and researchers. The first recorded use of "pinkeye" was "a contagious fever or influenza in the horse, so called for the color of the inflamed conjunctiva."[6] Pinkeye is a catchall term producers use to label diverse eye conditions of cattle. Similarly, IBK may be an "umbrella diagnosis"[7] by veterinarians who usually characterize IBK on history, signalment, and typical clinical signs of epiphora, ocular discharge, blepharospasm, conjunctivitis, and keratitis.[5] Some

Sydney School of Veterinary Science, The University of Sydney, Camden, NSW, Australia
E-mail address: pkne0185@uni.sydney.edu.au

Vet Clin Food Anim 37 (2021) 237–252
https://doi.org/10.1016/j.cvfa.2021.03.001
0749-0720/21/Crown Copyright © 2021 Published by Elsevier Inc. All rights reserved.

researchers additionally require isolation or detection of *Moraxella bovis* to define IBK cases.

M bovis, a gram-negative bacterium, is commonly considered the cause of IBK. Almost all IBK research has focused on *M bovis;* however, its role in IBK is not settled. Pathogenesis of field IBK may involve characteristics of *M bovis* and cofactors, like other organisms (including commensals), host response, and environment. IBK challenge studies routinely involve high doses of virulent (piliated and hemolytic) strains of *M bovis* introduced by unnatural routes or onto damaged corneas, either scarified or ultraviolet (UV) light irradiated, and be too contrived to resemble natural occurring disease.[8] *M bovis* may not be the sole cause of IBK. It is not known if *M bovis* is a necessary component of all IBK[9,10]; it could be a secondary opportunist[11] or even incidental, not causative.[10,12]

DEFINITION OF INFECTIOUS BOVINE KERATOCONJUNCTIVITIS

Lack of case definition means workers may not be describing the same disease.[7] This may hamper research syntheses efforts.

We propose IBK be defined as a herd disease of cattle with high morbidity (mean proportion affected more than 2% in calves and 0.6% in cows) and rapid spread (mean time course within herd of 30 days) of clinical signs restricted to the eye, including conjunctivitis and/or keratitis with a significant number (10% or more) developing corneal ulceration.

DIAGNOSIS OF INFECTIOUS BOVINE KERATOCONJUNCTIVITIS

Diagnosis is collection of evidence to categorize illness. Most ocular diseases have no pathognomonic (classically distinctive) clinical signs. Commonly cited clinical manifestations of IBK may be a clinical disguise worn by different bovine ocular diseases. A common error in disease diagnosis is using nondiscriminatory findings to support a diagnosis. It was reported that some animals with a "carrier form" of *M bovis* show intermittent or chronic excessive lacrimation,[13] and erosions of eyelid margins are seen occasionally in eyes chronically infected with *M bovis*[14]; however, using clinical signs alone it is not possible to distinguish IBK from other causes of keratoconjunctivitis.[5,15] As Penberthy[2] stated in 1897, *"symptoms shown are those usually exhibited in inflammation of these parts."* Thus, diagnosis of IBK, like other diseases, requires a combination of evidence collected from signalment, history, clinical signs, and/or laboratory diagnostics.

Signalment and History

Age, breed, and seasonality help narrow diagnostic focus, with young *Bos taurus* more frequently affected in warmer months.[5,13] IBK is an unlikely diagnosis in adult Zebu cattle in mid-winter. Other possible risk factors include periocular pigmentation, sunlight, flies, dust, pollens, wind, rough forage, nutritional deficiencies, and concurrent infections.[5,13,16]

Herd-Level Clinical Signs

Clinicians should be wary diagnosing IBK in an individual animal, as it is a herd disease.[17] IBK is an epizootic disease, that is, temporarily prevalent and widespread, affecting only the eyes, particularly of young *B taurus* in warmer seasons. Within-herd characteristics of IBK outbreaks, both portion of herd diseased and time course in herd, vary. Inconsistencies may be explained by differing disease definitions or interactions among host, agents, and environment.

Within-Herd Prevalence

Data on within-herd prevalence are limited and range widely, for example, from 1.1% to 57.0% to 98.0% in the United States (**Table 1**, Elliott J. Dennis and Mac Kneipp's article, "A Review of Global Prevalence and Economic Impacts of Infectious Bovine Keratoconjunctivitis," in this issue).[18] Using the main IBK risk factors of cattle subspecies, age, and geographic climate, estimated annual prevalence of IBK in subspecies *B taurus* is 10.00% (minimum 5.00, maximum 20.00) in calves and 3.00% (1.00, 5.00) in cows, and in *Bos indicus* 2.00% (1.00, 5.00) in calves and 0.60% (0.00, 2.00) in cows.[18] Estimates relate to a country's between-herd prevalence but are used here to define within-herd prevalence.

Time Course in Herd

IBK occurs in outbreaks and is described as highly contagious; however, there are few data on time course in a herd. What data are available on IBK duration mostly refer to disease in individuals measured in days to healing. IBK-affected eyes are reported to heal in 1 to 3 weeks but can recover at any stage, with most healing in 60 days.[19] A "simple" corneal ulcer, one that is not large, deep, or infected, may heal without attention within 4 to 7 days with time to healing linearly related to maximal ulcer size.[20] IBK ulcers are infected, therefore, by definition, "complicated," nonetheless IBK ulcers smaller than 5 mm in diameter often heal spontaneously.[17] Unsurprisingly, a systematic review of antibiotic treatments for IBK found treatment of many kinds improve healing times.[21] Thirteen suitable trials extracted in this review observed treatment response from 15 to 108 days. The study suggested the best time to observe a difference between treatments (using corneal ulcer area as outcome) is between day 7 and 10, and that beyond day 16 choice of antibiotic intervention or placebo makes no difference. Combining range of IBK time course in individuals and knowledge that IBK occurs seasonally, it is estimated the mean time course of IBK in a herd is 30 days (minimum 7, maximum 90).

One key issue of diagnosing IBK is it is assumed to be an infectious process; however, it remains unclear if there is transmission of virulent organism between cattle. Transmission studies are not conclusive. Anecdotally, it is suggested IBK cases increase if animals are gathered in yards and assumed this means "transmission" is occurring. However, conditions in the yard to cause IBK to "occur" in one animal also make it likely to occur in others, for example, flies, dust, ocular trauma. *M bovis* may be transmitted by flies to surfaces[16] but without some intervening factor, like flies or environmental insults, transmission by contact appears inconsequential.[22] Nonetheless, a common feature of IBK is a significant number of animals in the herd, typically 10% of *B taurus* and 2% *B indicus* calves and/or 3% *B taurus* and 0.6% *B indicus* cows, affected in a short period of time, typically 30 days or less.

The combination of typical clinical signs, a herd history of IBK, and high (more than 15% of calves in the herd) and rapid (occurring seasonally in spring) infectivity rate, are considered more reliable to characterize IBK than bacterial culture due to risk of opportunistic secondary infection.[8]

Individual-Level Clinical Signs

IBK affects primarily only the eyes of cattle. A lack of systemic involvement is a feature that helps differentiate IBK from other diseases with ocular signs, for example, conjunctivitis is significant but secondary in viral pneumonias, bluetongue, Rinderpest, besnoitiosis, bovine viral diarrhea, malignant catarrhal fever (MCF), and infectious bovine rhinotracheitis (IBR) caused by bovine herpesvirus type 1 (BHV-1).[23]

Table 1
Differential diagnoses of IBK

Disease	Ocular Signs	Systemic Signs	Herd Disease	Ref
IBK	✔	✗	✔	13,17
Ocular foreign body, trauma	✔ Acute fluorescein staining differs	✗	✔	5,37
Fly worry (*Musca autumnalis* [face fly] most studied)	✔ corneal ulcers unlikely	✗	✔	16,28
UV light exposure	✔	✗	✔	44,53
IBR (BHV-1) infection	✔ fewer corneal ulcers comorbidity?	✔ Mucosal erosions Respiratory Gastrointestinal	✔	25,54,55
Adenovirus infection	✔ less keratitis	✗	✔	15,26
Ocular squamous cell carcinoma	✔ similar initially	✗	✗	55
Mycoplasma spp infection	✔ conjunctivitis, comorbidity?	✔ Respiratory Arthritis Otitis	✔	23,52
Chlamydiosis	✔ conjunctivitis, less corneal ulcers	✔ variable multisystemic	✔ high morbidity, protracted course	23,36
Vitamin A deficiency	✔ profuse epiphora, corneal softening	✔ Night blindness other	✔ IBK risk factor?	27
MCF virus infection	✔ more chemosis, conjunctivitis, limbal corneal ulcers	✔ Mucosal erosions other	✗ unlikely	23,25,55
Listeriosis, bovine iritis, "silage eye"	✔ more uveitis	✔ variable multisystemic	✔ winter-spring, housed, feeder use	5
Thelazia (eyeworm)	✔ variable	✗	✗ unlikely	15
Phenothiazine (anthelmintic)	✔ corneal edema, keratitis	✗	Possible in calves recover without sun exposure	56
Congenital disorders: entropion, ectropion, pestivirus (BVDV) bluetongue- BTV-8	✔ less or no ulceration many are rare	✔ (some)	Possible	23

Pasteurella multocida (capsular type A) infection has been listed as an IBK differential.[23]

Clinical appearance of IBK-affected eyes is often repeated since Billings[1] in 1889 described "keratitis contagiosa" as *"an initial serous ocular discharge later becomes purulent and is followed by blepharitis and conjunctivitis. Around 3 days later cloudiness of the center of the cornea develops, this becomes more diffuse and the cornea thickens. In many cases the center of the cornea then becomes yellow and thins, the yellow spot is surrounded by white discolouration and blood vessels from the limbus are seen giving a red rim to the opaque cornea. The cornea sometimes ulcerates and even ruptures."* Such descriptions have little diagnostic value, as the ocular inflammatory response is limited and identical to different challenges (**Figs. 1** and **2**). There was dispute whether IBK was primarily a keratitis, a conjunctivitis, or if they occurred simultaneously,[24] and disparity of clinical features and order they occur was taken as proof IBK is more than one condition.[7] IBK-associated keratitis, defined as circumscribed, often centrally located, corneal ulceration, is the most definitive clinical sign of IBK, but it too is not pathognomonic.

Profuse lacrimation with epiphora is a typical initial sign but easily missed.[5] Ocular discharge with IBK is serous or mucopurulent, amount and type could indicate conjunctival or corneal involvement and nature of initiating agent (IBK discharge more than MCF but less than IBR[25]). However, no differences were clinically evident in keratoconjunctivitis caused by *M bovis* and adenovirus,[26] and there are other causes of bovine ocular discharge, such as vitamin A deficiency[27] and fly worry.[28] For some cattle, slight lacrimation appears normal, and with fly worry alone there are marked differences in tearing between breeds and individuals.[28]

Conjunctivitis is not a feature of every clinical IBK case and not specific; it can be caused by BHV-1, MCF virus,[25] bovine adenovirus,[26] mycoplasma, chlamydia,[23]

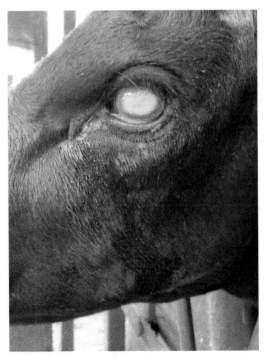

Fig. 1. Typical "pinkeye" may only be describing any complicated corneal ulcer left untreated (this eye has been fluorescein stained).

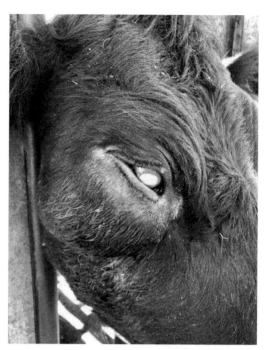

Fig. 2. "Pinkeye" caused by foreign body. A stick had penetrated the lateral cheek.

listeria,[5] *Mycoplasma bovoculi*,[29] injury, or occur secondarily, for example, to exposure keratitis and eyelid paralysis.[23] Attempts have been made to characterize bovine conjunctivitis by histology.[30] Blepharitis and matting of eyelashes can occur in IBK. *M bovoculi*–associated ulcerative blepharitis is reported.[29]

Many articles emphasize ulcerative keratitis as indicative of IBK. There are few infectious causes of primary keratitis, most prominent being herpesviruses, with *M bovis* described as the only bacteria of veterinary importance that can initiate corneal ulceration.[31] Corneal ulceration has been reported in *M bovis*–challenge studies of gnotobiotic[30,32] and conventional calves, housed to decrease predisposing factors (UV light, flies, dust, wind)[32] and with minimal or no evidence of other infections.[7] However, generally in such studies when IBK occurred it was mild compared with field IBK, suggesting it does not have a simple causative mechanism.[32] Standard *M bovis*–challenge models came to include corneal "preconditioning" (damage) by scarification or UV irradiation.[8]

The proposed entry point for *M bovis* is the corneal or conjunctival surface, with pili considered necessary virulence factors to adhere.[17,33] The normal description is central corneal opacity (corneal edema) developing before ulceration[13] that occurs within a few days, but may be delayed up to 2 weeks after onset of signs.[34] Early corneal lesions, or corneal vesicles, are small and easily missed.[17] Ulcers enlarge or small ulcers coalesce and deepen to involve the stroma, with accompanying corneal edema, and mild to moderate aqueous flare and iridocyclitis. Alternatively, IBK keratitis is described as a central, small, raised yellow-to-white corneal abscess that may slough leaving an ulcer.

Central corneal ulceration is noted as characteristic of IBK from earliest reports,[1] used to clinically differentiate IBK from IBR and MCF,[25] to define experimentally produced IBK, and as primary outcome in *M bovis*–challenge studies.[35] However, it does not occur in all cases of IBK. IBK may manifest as conjunctivitis only. Conjunctivitis without corneal involvement is counted in some IBK scores.[7] Corneal defects may occur initially in the peripheral cornea, including in *M bovis*–challenge of gnotobiotic calves.[30] Other ocular diseases can create a central lesion, including adenovirus.[26] Apparent central cornea involvement may sometimes be due to the ocular repair process. Peripheral lesions, close to the limbic blood supply, heal more rapidly than central ulcers remote from a blood supply.[20] So, although not all IBK may start in the central cornea, severe corneal injury normally heals last in the central cornea. The one gnotobiotic calf that developed central ulceration in the study by Rogers[30] exhibited the most severe IBK with hypopyon. IBK corneal scars often appear centrally located, but again this is not unique to IBK.[36]

Shape and fluorescein-staining characteristics of corneal ulcers may aid diagnosis.[20,37] IBK-associated ulcers are described as round-to-oval and deep.[25] Deep ulcers have less distinct (hazy) borders with fluorescein compared with shallow ulcers due to stain leaking into the stroma. It was reported that IBK ulceration is deepest at the center of the cornea,[38] unsurprisingly as bovine corneas are thickest (1.5 mm to 2.0 mm) centrally.

Corneal color and clarity (cloudiness) are indicators of ocular disease process much relied on in veterinary ophthalmology.[20] The hydrophilic stroma is sandwiched between and protected from liquid tear film and aqueous humor by waterproof epithelial and endothelial barriers, and maintained in active "deturgescence" (dehydration) by an ATPase sodium-potassium exchange pump.[39] Corneal edema appears blue, and if due to loss of epithelial barrier, like in IBK, it will be focal because the ATPase pump remains active. Stroma is exposed and takes up fluorescein. By comparison, endothelial barrier breach results in diffuse blue edema and fluorescein is not taken up.

IBK scars are commonly referred to as "blue eye," but on close inspection, the corneal color is gray or dull white. Although blue indicates active corneal edema, white indicates corneal fibrosis of healing or healed insults. During repair of stromal injuries collagen laid down results in these gray-white opacities or scars. The difference between blue and white corneal lesions is subtle but important; therefore, it is worthwhile to use good ophthalmology technique, including dim ambient light, bright focal light source, and magnification, to help differentiate (**Figs. 3–5**). Cattle producers may treat inappropriately if they cannot differentiate active IBK from corneal scarring[17] (**Figs. 6–8**). However, little is straightforward with this disease syndrome, and IBK-affected eyes may have more than 1 corneal color, as damage is often a combination of edema (blue), vascularization (red), pus (greenish-yellow), and repair (gray-white) (**Figs. 9 and 10**).

With severe corneal damage, blood vessels may enter the avascular cornea to deliver a fuller inflammatory response. The position and form of corneal vessels indicates location, depth, and timeline of an injury.[20] Type of leukocytes recruited and humoral immunoglobulin response pattern give insights into ocular disease etiology, but there are few such studies relating to IBK.[7,40] With corneal vascularization, ulcer repair is well-advanced in 2 to 3 weeks and complete in 1 to 2 months. Bovine corneas appear more robust than those of dogs and horses, with remarkable capacity for repair, particularly in calves.[25] Nonetheless, IBK may cause permanent corneal scar characterized as nebula, macula, and leukoma, being minor, moderate, and notable opacity, respectively.[20] IBK can lead to descemetocele and perforated cornea,[25] most retain globe shape[13] but some progress to buphthalmia (popeye) or phthisis bulbi (small shrunken globe) (**Fig. 11**). Blindness caused by IBK, whether partial or complete, temporary or permanent, is an animal welfare and workplace safety issue.

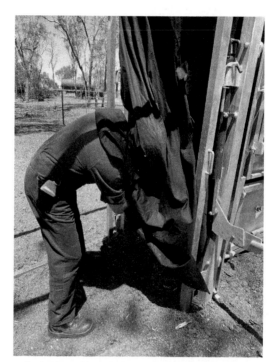

Fig. 3. Dark sheet to diminish ambient light and aid ocular examination.

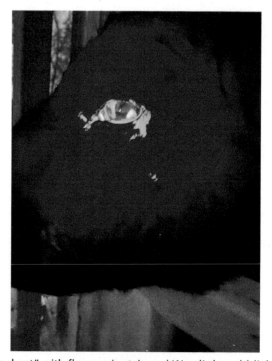

Fig. 4. "Under the sheet" with fluorescein stain and Wood's (*purple*) light.

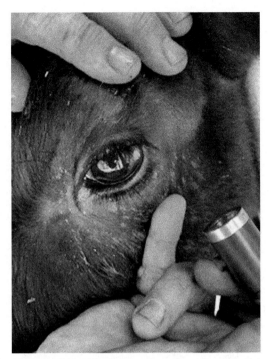

Fig. 5. Corneal ulcer more visible with fluorescein stain and purple light.

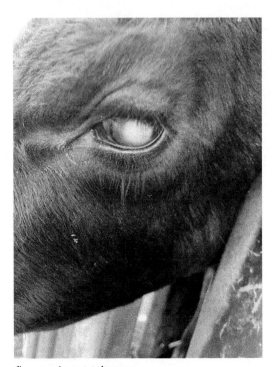

Fig. 6. Corneal scar-fluorescein not taken up.

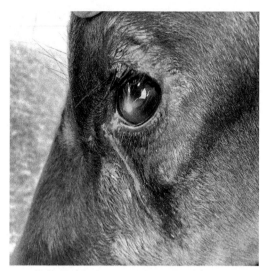

Fig. 7. Active corneal ulcer-corneal edema (*blue*), fluorescein taken up with hazy edges and epiphora.

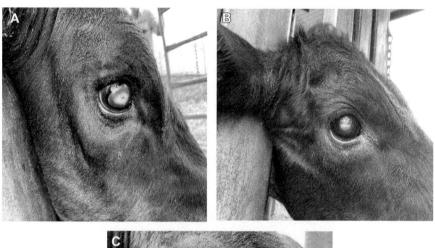

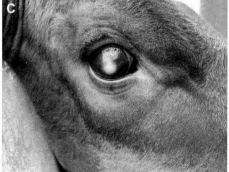

Fig. 8. (*A–C*) Three eyes with corneal scars; note no tear staining on face.

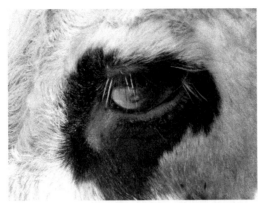

Fig. 9. Multiple corneal colors: corneal sequestrum ("scab"), descemetocele, and vascularization.

Loss of value due to ocular scarring is one of the major commercial losses associated with IBK.[18]

Clinical signs of keratitis include pain witnessed as lacrimation, blepharospasm, and photophobia. Moraxella keratitis in humans is typically painless,[41] but in an experiment involving corneal scarification with or without *M bovis* inoculation, calves showed greatly increased photophobia and blepharospasm with IBK-associated corneal ulcerations compared with scarification alone.[42] Using signs of ocular pain for diagnosis and prognosis in corneal disease is problematic. In mammalian species, the cornea is the most densely innervated area of the body surface, with most nerve endings located superficially in the epithelium, meaning superficial keratitis is more painful than deeper injury. Clinicians should be wary using pain to interpret success of therapy, as diminishing pain could mean a deepening ulcer.[20]

Laboratory Diagnostics

The most used laboratory test to confirm a diagnosis of IBK, microbiological culture from ocular swabs, is problematic because *M bovis*[43,44] (and *Mycoplasma bovoculi*[45]) may be cultured from healthy cattle, and there is risk of rapid invasion by secondary

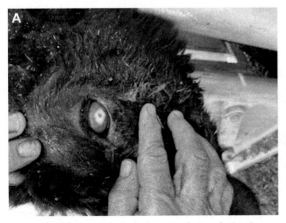
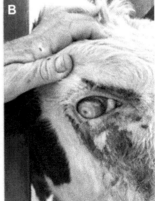

Fig. 10. (*A*, *B*) Deep central ulcers and vascularization.

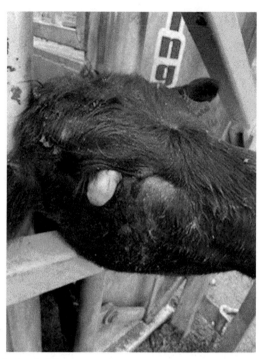

Fig. 11. Buphthalmia (popeye).

organisms,[8,46] sample contamination,[17] and involvement of other causally associated and potential confounder organisms (including *Mycoplasma bovoculi, Mycoplasma bovis,* and BHV-1).[47,48]

Because of difficulty differentiating pathogens, especially *Moraxella, Neisseria,* and *Branhamella* spp,[49] using early techniques like stains and microscopic identification, culture characteristics and biochemical profile, alternative methods were sought. *M bovis* antibodies were demonstrated in cattle sera after natural and experimental infection, however cattle (and mice) did not always develop antibodies.[50] Researchers, unable to demonstrate systemic antibodies, suggested immune response could be localized to lacrimal secretions. Studies found immune response, both systemic immunoglobulin G and local immunoglobulin A, was short-lived.[51] Enzyme-linked immunosorbent assay and fluorescent antibody tests[44] for anti-*M bovis* antibodies are described. More recently, molecular techniques, polymerase chain reaction (PCR) assay, and 16S ribosomal RNA microbial community sequencing analysis, have been used in IBK, but so far failed to clarify the role of *M bovis* and other pathogens.[10,47,52] PCR assay detected organisms from tears more frequently and reported more than 1 organism more often than culture.[47] A multiplex real-time PCR panel assay was highly sensitive and specific for detection and differentiation of 5 IBK-associated pathogens; *M bovis, Moraxella bovoculi, Mycoplasma bovis, Mycoplasma bovoculi,* and BHV-1.[48]

CLINICAL SUBCLASSIFICATION AND INFECTIOUS BOVINE KERATOCONJUNCTIVITIS SCORES

Researchers have subclassified IBK and produced IBK scores. IBK scores are prone to bias, for example, the score devised by George and colleagues[57] and used by others assumes all epiphora is a sign of IBK. Although digital photography and machine learning may improve IBK scores, because IBK-associated ocular changes are not unique, rather than devising novel scores, IBK-affected eyes should be characterized with the 4 standard ophthalmic descriptors used for ocular disease in other species. Specifically, by describing (in order) any of the following:

1. *Conjunctival disease* by presence of hyperemia, swelling, chemosis, amount and type of discharge
2. *Corneal disease* as acute or chronic, ulcerative (size, depth, shape, fluorescein-staining properties) or nonulcerative, plus any corneal vascularization and color
3. *Other ocular involvement*, for example, iridocyclitis, iridospasm, buphthalmia, phthisis bulbi, loss of sight
4. *Signs of pain*: blepharospasm, photophobia, lacrimation, and behavior changes

SUMMARY

Cattle are subject to many different ocular diseases. To ensure all are describing the same disease, clear concise case definitions are required. Although the term "pinkeye" might be used by producers, we would encourage veterinarians to describe ocular lesions by precise ophthalmic terms; for example, keratitis, conjunctivitis, keratoconjunctivitis. We propose that the term "infectious bovine keratoconjunctivitis (IBK)" be reserved for herd disease affecting only eyes with high morbidity (mean proportion affected more than 2% in calves and 0.6% in cows) and rapid dissemination (mean time course within herd of 30 days) of acute keratoconjunctivitis, signs of which may include increased lacrimation, epiphora, serous or mucopurulent conjunctivitis, and, most significantly, keratitis, seen initially as focal corneal edema (blue) and without intervention ≥10% developing fluorescein-positive corneal ulceration, which would typically when mature be deep (hazy), circumscribed, oval-shaped, and paracentral.

"Ocular moraxellosis" is bovine keratoconjunctivitis from which *Moraxella* spp are demonstrated.

CLINICS CARE POINTS

- Veterinary clinicians should avoid the term 'pinkeye' and use precise ophthalmology terms to accurately describe ocular lesions of cattle.
- Clinical diagnosis of infectious bovine keratoconjunctivitis requires a combination of evidence from signalment, history, clinical signs and/or laboratory diagnostics.
- Infectious bovine keratoconjunctivitis is an acute herd disease affecting only the eyes with high morbidity and rapid spread, the most significant clinical sign is corneal ulceration.
- Accurate disease diagnoses and description is essential for appropriate management.

DISCLOSURE

The author has nothing to disclose.

REFERENCES

1. Billings F. Keratitis contagiosa in cattle. Bull Agric Exp Station Nebr 1889;3: 247–52.

2. Penberthy JE. Contagious ophthalmia in cattle. J Compend Pathol Ther 1897;10: 263–4.
3. Poels J. Keratitis infectiosa der Runderen (keratitis polybacillosa). Tijdschr Veeartsenijk 1911;38:758–66.
4. Burns MJ, O'Connor AM. Assessment of methodological quality and sources of variation in the magnitude of vaccine efficacy: a systematic review of studies from 1960 to 2005 reporting immunization with *Moraxella bovis* vaccines in young cattle. Vaccine 2008;26:144–52.
5. Alexander D. Infectious bovine keratoconjunctivitis: a review of cases in clinical practice. Vet Clin North Am 2010;26:487–503.
6. The Oxford English Dictionary. In: Simpson JA, Weiner ESC, editors. The Oxford English Dictionary. 2nd edition. Oxford: Clarendon Press; 1989. p. 873.
7. Aikman JG, Allan EM, Selman IE. Experimental production of infectious bovine keratoconjunctivitis. Vet Rec 1985;117:234–9.
8. O'Connor A, Cooper V, Censi L, et al. A 2-year randomized blinded controlled trial of a conditionally licensed Moraxella bovoculi vaccine to aid in prevention of infectious bovine keratoconjunctivitis in Angus beef calves. J Vet Intern Med 2019; 33(6):2786–93.
9. O'Connor AM. Infectious Bovine Keratoconjunctivitis Management. American Association of Bovine Practitioners Annual Conference, September 20-22, 2007, Vancouver, British Columbia. p. 66-70.
10. Cullen JN, Lithio A, Seetharam AS, et al. Microbial community sequencing analysis of the calf eye microbiota and relationship to infectious bovine keratoconjunctivitis. Vet Microbiol 2017;207:267–79.
11. Prieto C, Serra DO, Martina P, et al. Evaluation of biofilm-forming capacity of *Moraxella bovis*, the primary causative agent of infectious bovine keratoconjuntivitis. Vet Microbiol 2013;166:504–15.
12. O'Connor AM, Brace S, Gould S, et al. A randomized clinical trial evaluating a farm-of-origin autogenous *Moraxella bovis* vaccine to control infectious bovine keratoconjunctivitis (Pinkeye) in beef cattle. J Vet Intern Med 2011;25:1447–53.
13. Brown MH, Brightman AH, Fenwick BW, et al. Infectious bovine keratoconjunctivitis: a review. J Vet Intern Med 1998;12:259–66.
14. Huntington PJ, Coloe PJ, Bryden JD, et al. Isolation of *Moraxella* sp from horses with conjunctivitis. Aust Vet J 1987;64:118–9.
15. Wilcox GE. The aetiology of infectious bovine keratoconjunctivitis in Queensland. 1. *Moraxella bovis*. Aust Vet J 1970;46:409–14.
16. Hall RD. Relationship of the face fly (Diptera: Muscidae) to pinkeye in cattle: a review and synthesis of the relevant literature12. J Med Entomol 1984;21:361–5.
17. Angelos JA. Infectious bovine keratoconjunctivitis (pinkeye). Vet Clin North Am Food Anim Pract 2015;31:61–79.
18. Dennis EJ, Kneipp M. A review of global prevalence and economic impacts of infectious bovine keratoconjunctivitis. Vet Clin North Am 2012;37(2):237–52.
19. George LW, Wilson WD, Baggot JD, et al. Antibiotic treatment of *Moraxella bovis* infection in cattle. J Am Vet Med Assoc 1984;185:1206–9.
20. Maggs DJ. Diseases Cornea and Sclera. In: Maggs DJ, Miller PE, Ofri R, editors. Slatter's Fundamentals of veterinary ophthalmology. 6th ed. St Louis (MO): Elsevier; 2018. p. 213–53.
21. Cullen JN, Yuan C, Totton S, et al. A systematic review and meta-analysis of the antibiotic treatment for infectious bovine keratoconjunctivitis: an update. Anim Health Res Rev 2016;17:60–75.

22. Kopecky KE, Pugh GW, McDonald TJ. Infectious bovine keratoconjunctivitis: contact transmission. Am J Vet Res 1986;47:622–6.
23. Constable PD. In: Veterinary medicine : a textbook of the diseases of cattle, horses, sheep, pigs and goats. 11th edition. St Louis (MO): Elsevier; 2017.
24. Wilcox GE. Infectious bovine kerato-conjunctivitis: a review. Vet Bull 1968;38: 349–60.
25. Rankin AJ, Sutton GA. Livestock ophthalmology. In: Maggs DJ, Miller PE, Ofri R, editors. Slatter's Fundamentals of veterinary ophthalmology. 6th edition. St Louis (MO): Elsevier; 2018. p. 471–95.
26. Wilcox GE. The aetiology of infectious bovine keratoconjunctivitis in Queensland 2. Adenovirus. Aust Vet J 1970;46:415–20.
27. McDowell LR. Vitamin A. Vitamins in animal and human nutrition. 2nd edition. Ames (IA): Iowa State University Press; 2000. p. 15–90.
28. Shugart JI, Campbell DB, Hudson DB, et al. Ability of face fly to cause damage to eyes of cattle. J Econ Entomol 1979;72:633–5.
29. Galvão KN, Angelos JA. Ulcerative blepharitis and conjunctivitis in adult dairy cows and association with *Moraxella bovoculi*. Can Vet J 2010;51:400.
30. Rogers DG. Pathogenesis of corneal and conjunctival lesions caused by *Moraxella bovis* in Gnotobiotic calves. *Veterinary Science*. Ames (IA): Iowa State University; 1987.
31. Maggs DJ. Cornea and Sclera. In: Maggs DJ, Miller PE, Ofri R, editors. Slatter's Fundamentals of veterinary ophthalmology. 4th edition. St Louis (MO): Saunders, Elsevier; 2008. p. 170–202.
32. Chandler RL, Turfrey BA, Smith K, et al. Virulence of *Moraxella bovis* in gnotobiotic calves. Vet Rec 1980;106:364–5.
33. Lepper AWD. Vaccination against infectious bovine keratoconjunctivitis: protective efficacy and antibody response induced by pili of homologous and heterologous strains of *Moraxella bovis*. Aust Vet J 1988;65:310–6.
34. Smith JA, George LW. Treatment of acute ocular *Moraxella bovis* infections in calves with parenterally administered long-acting oxytetracyline formulation. Am J Vet Res 1985;46:804–7.
35. Gould S, Dewell R, Tofflemire K, et al. Randomized blinded challenge study to assess association between *Moraxella bovoculi* and infectious bovine keratoconjunctivitis in dairy calves. Vet Microbiol 2013;164:108–15.
36. Otter A, Twomey DF, Rowe NS, et al. Suspected chlamydial keratoconjunctivitis in British cattle. Vet Rec 2003;152:787–8.
37. Angelos JA, Gohary KG, Ball LM, et al. Randomized controlled field trial to assess efficacy of a *Moraxella bovis* pilin-cytotoxin–*Moraxella bovoculi* cytotoxin subunit vaccine to prevent naturally occurring infectious bovine keratoconjunctivitis. Am J Vet Res 2012;73:1670–5.
38. Weech GM, Renshaw HW. Infectious bovine keratoconjunctivitis: bacteriologic, immunologic and clinical responses of cattle to experimental exposure with *Moraxella bovis*. Comp Immunol Microbiol Infect Dis 1983;6:81–94.
39. Wilcock BP. General pathology of the eye. In: Maggs DJ, Miller PE, Ofri R, editors. Slatter's fundamentals of veterinary ophthalmology. 4th edition. St Louis (MO): Saunders Elsevier; 2008. p. 62–80.
40. Arora AK. Host parasite relationship as it affects the epizootiology of bovine infectious keratoconjunctivitis. Veterinary medical science. Urbana (IL): University of Illinois; 1973. p. 135.
41. Barash A, Chou TY. Moraxella atlantae keratitis presenting with an infectious ring ulcer. Am J Ophthalmol case Rep 2017;7:62–5.

42. Dewell RD, Millman ST, Gould SA, et al. Evaluating approaches to measuring ocular pain in bovine calves with corneal scarification and infectious bovine keratoconjunctivitis–associated corneal ulcerations. J Anim Sci 2014;92:1161–72.
43. Zbrun MV, Zielinski GC, Piscitelli HC, et al. Dynamics of *Moraxella bovis* infection and humoral immune response to bovine herpes virus type 1 during a natural outbreak of infectious bovine keratoconjunctivitis in beef calves. J Vet Sci 2011; 12:347–52.
44. Lepper AWD, Barton IJ. Infectious bovine keratoconjunctivitis: seasonal variation in cultural, biochemical and immunoreactive properties of *Moraxella bovis* isolated from the eyes of cattle. Aust Vet J 1987;64:33–9.
45. Angelos JA. *Moraxella bovoculi* and infectious bovine keratoconjunctivitis: cause or coincidence? Vet Clin North Am: Food Anim Pract 2010;26:73–8.
46. Cullen JN, Engelken TJ, Cooper V, et al. Randomized blinded controlled trial to assess the association between a commercial vaccine against *Moraxella bovis* and the cumulative incidence of infectious bovine keratoconjunctivitis in beef calves. J Am Vet Med Assoc 2017;251:345–51.
47. O'Connor AM, Shen HG, Wang C, et al. Descriptive epidemiology of *Moraxella bovis, Moraxella bovoculi* and *Moraxella ovis* in beef calves with naturally occurring infectious keratoconjunctivitis (Pinkeye). Vet Microbiol 2012;155:374–80.
48. Zheng W, Porter E, Noll L, et al. A multiplex real-time PCR assay for the detection and differentiation of five bovine pinkeye pathogens. J Microbiol Methods 2019; 160:87–92.
49. Pedersen KB. Isolation and description of a haemolytic species of *Neisseria* (*N. ovis*) from cattle with infectious keratoconjunctivitis. Acta Pathol Microbiol Scand 1972;80(1):135–9.
50. Pugh JGW, Hughes DE. Infectious bovine keratoconjunctivitis induced by different experimental methods. Cornell Vet 1971;61:23.
51. di Girolamo FA, Sabatini DJ, Fasan RA, et al. Evaluation of cytokines as adjuvants of infectious bovine keratoconjunctivitis vaccines. Vet Immunol Immunopathol 2012;145:563–6.
52. Schnee C, Heller M, Schubert E, et al. Point prevalence of infection with *Mycoplasma bovoculi* and *Moraxella* spp. in cattle at different stages of infectious bovine keratoconjunctivitis. Vet J 2015;203:92–6.
53. Hughes DE, Pugh JGW, McDonald TJ. Experimental bovine infectious keratoconjunctivitis caused by sunlamp irradiation and *Moraxella bovis* infection: determination of optimal irradiation. Am J Vet Res 1968;29:821–7.
54. Hughes JP, Olander HJ, Wada M. Keratoconjunctivitis associated with infectious bovine rhinotracheitis. J Am Vet Med Assoc 1964;145:32–9.
55. George LW. Clinical infectious bovine keraotconjunctivitis. Compend Contin Educ 1984;6:712–22.
56. Townsend WM. Food & fibre-producing animal ophthalmology. In: Gelatt KN, editor. Essentials of veterinary ophthalmology. Oxford, England: ProQuest Ebook Central: Wiley; 2013. p. 384–90.
57. George LW, Mihalyi J, Edmondson A, et al. Topically applied furazolidone or parenterally administered oxytetracycline for the treatment of infectious bovine keratoconjunctivtis. J Am Vet Med Assoc 1988;192:1415–22.

Bovine Immune Responses to *Moraxella bovis* and *Moraxella bovoculi* Following Vaccination and Natural or Experimental Infections

John A. Angelos, DVM, PhD, DACVIM[a],*, Paola Elizalde, DVM[b],
Philip Griebel, DVM, PhD[b,c]

KEYWORDS

- Commensal bacteria • IgA antibody • IgG antibody
- Infectious bovine keratoconjunctivitis (IBK) • *Moraxella bovis* • *Moraxella bovoculi*
- Mucosal immunity • Systemic immunity

KEY POINTS

- Pilin and cytotoxin (hemolysin) antigens and whole-cell bacterins have been reported to provide some protection against IBK in experimental and natural challenge settings.
- Fully protective *Moraxella* spp antigens against IBK have yet to be clearly defined.
- Whether bovine mucosal immune responses to *Moraxella* spp antigens are more beneficial for protection against IBK than systemic immune responses is not well understood.

INTRODUCTION

Over many years of vaccine research to develop effective infectious bovine keratoconjunctivitis (IBK) vaccines, different antigens, adjuvants, and routes of vaccination have been investigated. This article begins with an overview of bovine ocular immune responses, linkages between nasal and ocular immunity, and the roles that IgG and IgA may play in relation to IBK protection. Recent evidence that *Moraxella* spp reside as commensals in the upper respiratory tract (URT) and eye is also discussed, along with knowledge gaps regarding host-microbe interactions in young animals. Systemic and mucosal immune responses to *Moraxella* spp antigens are then discussed and evidence for protective or harmful immune responses against *Moraxella* spp antigens are considered.

[a] Department of Medicine and Epidemiology, School of Veterinary Medicine, University of California, Davis, CA, USA; [b] School of Public Health, University of Saskatchewan, Saskatoon, Saskatchewan, Canada; [c] VIDO-Intervac, University of Saskatchewan, Saskatoon, Saskatchewan, Canada
* Corresponding author.
E-mail address: jaangelos@ucdavis.edu

Vet Clin Food Anim 37 (2021) 253–266
https://doi.org/10.1016/j.cvfa.2021.03.002   **vetfood.theclinics.com**
0749-0720/21/© 2021 Elsevier Inc. All rights reserved.

OVERVIEW OF BOVINE OCULAR IMMUNE RESPONSES
Ocular Defenses Against Infection

The bovine eye is exposed to physical damage, foreign material, and pathogenic microorganisms that can irritate the ocular mucosa; such environmental factors have all been implicated in the pathogenesis of IBK. Innate and adaptive immune defense mechanisms are active in the bovine eye, however, and can help minimize the effects of ocular damage and control bacterial colonization. The conjunctival-associated lymphoid tissue (CALT) functions to sample and respond to foreign material and microorganisms, while minimizing inflammatory responses that could destroy ocular integrity and function.[1] Understanding CALT development and function is important for understanding IBK pathogenesis and may be important for the design of vaccines able to control colonization by *Moraxella* spp without exacerbating ocular damage. Ocular defense mechanisms are reviewed and discussed within the context of recent information that *Moraxella* spp reside as commensals in the URT[2] and eye[3] of young healthy calves.

Innate Immune Defenses

The ocular mucosal barrier consists of several important components, including the tear film, mucosal epithelium, and organized and diffuse lymphoid tissue. The tear film of mammals is organized in a trilaminar structure consisting of a lipid, aqueous, and mucin layer.[4] Meibomian glands produce the lipid layer and the lacrimal glands and the third eyelid produce the aqueous layer.[4] Goblets cells are responsible for production of mucins, including the gel-forming mucin-5AC (MUC5AC) and mucin-2 (MUC2), which are important proteins in the mucin layer of the tear film in humans and other mammals.[5] The bovine tear film has not been well characterized but a recent study confirmed expression of nine bovine membrane-associated mucins genes, including MUC5AC and MUC2, at enteric mucosal surfaces.[6]

Cattle possess a dorsal lacrimal gland, superior glands of the third eyelid, and the Harderian glands.[7] Lacrimal glands are considered part of the secretory immune system and the dorsal lacrimal gland is the main secretor of tears in cattle.[4,7] In cattle, the dorsal lacrimal gland is responsible for approximately 60% of the aqueous component of the tear film and 40% is contributed by the accessory lacrimal gland of the third eyelid. Antibody secreting plasma cells localize to the lacrimal glands and are an important source of the IgA secreted in tears,[8] which is the predominant antibody type present in bovine ocular secretions.[9] Following natural or experimental *Moraxella bovis* infection, calves develop increased levels of *Moraxella*-specific IgA in tears,[10] but the immune induction site for *Moraxella*-specific IgA B cells (also known as B lymphocytes) and subsequent homing of these *Moraxella*-specific IgA plasma cells (also known as plasma B cells) to specific sites within the eye has not been characterized.

Proteins and peptides in the tear film serve a variety of functions, including antimicrobial activity and the recruitment and activation of leukocytes.[8] Dust, microorganisms, or foreign material suspended in the tear film leave the eye through the lacrimal duct and are sampled by the lacrimal duct–associated lymphoid tissue. In cattle, the lacrimal drainage system is continuous with the conjunctiva via the lacrimal puncta and canaliculi located in the lacrimal sac and nasal secretions drain into the nose through the nasolacrimal duct.[8] Thus, environmental factors, such as wind and dust, that disrupt the integrity of the tear film may compromise ocular defenses against colonizing bacteria and compromise the recruitment and activation of immune cells required to respond to the ocular microbial community.

The conjunctiva is an epithelial surface characterized by lymphoid and nonlymphoid regions. In adult cattle, CALT is located primarily in the lower conjunctiva but is also present in the upper conjunctiva.[11] The nonlymphoid conjunctiva consists of stratified squamous epithelium that contains goblet cells.[11] The conjunctiva is also an important source of antimicrobial peptides and numerous dendritic cells (DCs) are present at the basal epithelial layer with processes that extend into the epithelial layer.[12] Despite the variety of innate immune defenses protecting the eye, analysis of the ocular microbiome of healthy calves identified a wide variety of resident bacteria, including *Moraxella* spp.[3]

The Adaptive Immune System

Organized lymphoid tissue in the conjunctiva is composed of either solitary or aggregated lymphoid follicles and specialized follicles-associated epithelium. Electron microscopic studies of bovine CALT revealed some follicles-associated epithelium cells have short and irregular apical microfolds and display morphologic similarities to M cells that can efficiently transcytose particulate material to underlying lymphoid tissue.[11] Thus, CALT follicles-associated epithelium may have the capacity to transport particulate material, such as bacteria, from the lower conjunctival sac to the underlying lymphoid follicles. The abundance of DCs within the conjunctival epithelium also suggests that if the integrity of the conjunctival epithelium is disrupted then bacterial antigens may be sampled and transported by DCs to the draining lymph node. It is unknown, however, when CALT and lacrimal duct–associated lymphoid tissue develop in young calves and at what age secretory IgA production begins in tears (**Table 1**). Therefore, it remains to be determined whether young calves are susceptible to IBK because of a limited capacity to produce a local IgA response following *Moraxella* spp colonization of the eye.

Table 1
Knowledge gaps in the understanding of bovine ocular immunity relevant to *Moraxella* spp colonization and control of IBK

Knowledge Gap	Relevance
Knowledge of when CALT development and function begins in calves	This information would enable one to know when IgA production begins in tears and is critical information for determining time of vaccine delivery and understanding capacity of the eye to respond to *Moraxella* spp colonization of the eye.
Knowledge of when *Moraxella* spp colonize the eye	This information would enable one to know if there is endogenous production of *Moraxella*-specific IgA in tears or if the induction of regulatory T cells blocks a local antibody response.
Knowledge if IgA B cells induced in nasal-associated lymphoid tissue can migrate to the lacrimal glands and conjunctival epithelium	This information would provide evidence whether IgA responses to commensal *Moraxella* spp in the URT or IgA responses to intranasal vaccines can influence the level of IgA antibody secreted in tears.
Knowledge of T-helper or T-regulatory cell induction in CALT	This would allow a better understanding of whether T-cell responses play an important role in controlling *Moraxella* spp colonization of the eye, and ocular pathology associated with IBK.

CD4 T lymphocytes are also located in the lower parts of the lymphoid follicles, the interfollicular region, and subepithelial regions of bovine CALT.[11] CD4 T-helper cells are critical for differentiation of antigen-specific IgA B cells, but CD4 T cells may also include regulatory T cells that down-regulate acquired immune responses.[13] It remains to be determined whether regulatory T cells specific for *Moraxella* spp are induced in CALT or possibly recruited to the eye from the URT (see **Table 1**) where *Moraxella* spp also reside as part of the commensal microbiome.[2] Further investigations are required to determine if antibody and T-cell responses contribute to the control of *Moraxella* spp colonization and IBK (see **Table 1**).

Links Between Nasal and Ocular Immune Systems

Although little is known about CALT development and ocular immune competence in neonatal calves, much more is known about the development of nasal-associated lymphoid tissue. Development of bovine nasal-associated lymphoid tissue, such as the nasopharyngeal tonsil, begins in utero and there is a rapid increase in the size and cellularity of this lymphoid tissue during the first 2 weeks after birth.[14] Rapid postnatal development of nasal-associated lymphoid tissue occurs in healthy calves and is thought to be driven by immune responses to commensal microflora. A recent study confirmed that secretory IgA responses to *Mannheimia haemolytica* and *Pasteurella multocida*, two URT commensal bacteria, are detected in nasal secretions of healthy newborn calves within 2 to 3 weeks after birth.[15] This early onset of secretory IgA responses is consistent with bacteria colonizing the URT within the first week of life.[2] A similar pattern was observed for the production of secretory IgA reacting with *M bovis* and *Moraxella bovoculi* when nasal secretions from neonatal calves were analyzed with whole bacterial cell enzyme-linked immunosorbent assay (ELISA) (Elizalde and Griebel, unpublished observations, 2020).

CALT development and function has not been studied in young calves and the onset of IgA antibody responses to the ocular microbiome, including *Moraxella* spp, has not been analyzed (see **Table 1**). The bovine ocular microbiome was analyzed in suckling beef calves, but the animals' age when sampled was not reported.[3] Thus, it is not known if *Moraxella* spp colonization of the eye lags behind colonization of the URT, but polymerase chain reaction analysis of ocular swabs from 8 to 12 week old dairy calves identified only 2 of 31 animals with *M bovis* DNA and one of 31 animals with *M bovoculi* DNA.[16] Delayed colonization of the eye by *Moraxella* spp may also result in delayed production of IgA in tears, but it is not known if IgA B cells induced in the neonatal URT may home to the lacrimal glands, supporting IgA secretion in tears. Determining the kinetics of *Moraxella* spp colonization of the eye and the onset of local IgA and T-cell responses is critical for developing reproducible models of IBK caused by *M bovis* and *M bovoculi*. IgA responses to *M bovis* pili were detected in ocular secretions collected from healthy 4- to 7-month-old beef calves before vaccination.[17] Disease models, especially those used to evaluate vaccines, require the use of naive animals that can be consistently infected and develop clinical disease.[18] This may be difficult to achieve when developing IBK models that use opportunistic pathogens that are members of the commensal microbiome if the bacteria have previously been recognized by the mucosal and systemic immune system.

IMMUNE RESPONSES TO *MORAXELLA* ANTIGENS
Parenterally Administered Moraxella bovis Bacterins

Multiple studies have demonstrated that cattle vaccinated parenterally with various *M bovis* preparations develop precipitating serum antibody responses directed against

M bovis antigens. Most reports have used dairy or beef calves between about 2 and 10 months of age. Tested antigens have included viable,[19,20] heat-killed,[20] and formalin killed[20–22] *M bovis*. As expected, vaccination with viable *M bovis* cultures caused anaphylactoid reactions in some vaccinates.[19] Reported benefits from whole *M bovis* cell-derived vaccines (but not a heat-killed *M bovis* vaccine[20]) included reduced colonization rates by *M bovis*,[19] and protection against IBK[21,22] following experimental challenge using an irradiation model of IBK. Following experimentally induced IBK in four 1- to 2-week-old calves, serum IgG specific for *M bovis* whole-cell and soluble antigens could be detected by ELISA.[23] Tear samples collected from IBK-affected calves in that study also had measurable increases in IgA directed at a whole cell *M bovis* antigen, but not to a solubilized *M bovis* antigen. This study underscored the importance of the antigen type used in immune-based assays for detecting antigen-specific immunoglobulins.

A large multicenter study, using a whole-cell *Quillaja* bark (QuilA)-adjuvanted bacterin that contained pilin and corneal degrading enzyme antigens, was conducted in approximately 5000 3- to 6-week-old calves.[24,25] In that study calves were vaccinated subcutaneously (SC) once or twice (approximate 3-week booster interval); control animals received no vaccination. The study evaluated outcomes following natural (field study) and experimental challenge (topical administration of *M bovis* placed under the third eyelid). The field study tested single (n = 1520 calves) or two (n = 1536 calves) doses of vaccine, and there were 1931 nonvaccinated control animals. Bacterial agglutination and ELISA were used to quantify serum antibody responses. This study reported no significant difference in bacterial agglutination titers among the three groups of field study calves; however, serum antibody responses measured by ELISA were higher in experimentally challenged cattle that received bacterins with the highest enzyme antigen activity. Vaccination in field study calves reduced the incidence of IBK following one (66 IBK cases) or two doses of vaccine (48 IBK cases) compared with control subjects (217 IBK cases). Limitations of this study include lack of reported blinding of investigators as to vaccines administered or randomization.

Mucosally Administered Moraxella bovis Bacterins

Two of the earliest studies that investigated mucosal vaccination for *M bovis* evaluated vaccines administered by aerosolizing 1 mL *M bovis* cultures to cows and calves using an atomizer.[26,27] Although details of the exact composition of the vaccine and delivery method were not provided, the *M bovis* strains were apparently piliated strains. The vaccine reportedly reduced IBK and resulted in less clinically severe disease in vaccinates. However, neither nasal secretion nor tear antibody responses were described in these studies and dams of vaccinated calves also received vaccination prepartum that may have elevated maternally derived anti-*M bovis* IgG antibody levels in calves.

Parenterally Administered Moraxella bovis Pili and Piliated Moraxella bovis Bacterins

The results of an investigation into different methods for preparing a native pilin vaccine showed that serum antipilin precipitating antibodies could be detected more often in 2- to 4-month-old dairy calves receiving SC-administered oil-based vaccines made with Freund incomplete adjuvant (FIA) compared with water-based pilin vaccines.[28] Although sample sizes in this study were small, compared with unvaccinated control calves, pilin-FIA vaccinated calves experienced lower rates of colonization with *M bovis* and IBK following experimental challenge. A subsequent study reported that a native *M bovis* pili vaccine mixed with diphtheria-tetanus-toxoid-pertussis vaccine (two SC doses, 21 days apart) enhanced serum precipitating antibody responses to pili and reduced the occurrence of IBK in homologous challenged beef and dairy calves.[29] Subconjunctival and SC administration of a native pilin vaccine administered with diphtheria-tetanus-toxoid-pertussis vaccine as a two-dose series 14 days apart was also reported to protect calves against experimental homologous challenge.[30]

A vaccine made of *M bovis* pilin adjuvanted with 25% aluminum hydroxide administered intramuscularly and boostered on Day 28 protected dairy calves following experimental challenge approximately 2 and 3.5 weeks postvaccination.[31] Vaccinated calves had reduced clinical lesion scores and high serum antipilin IgG responses. Importantly, this study provided quantitative information on the antigenic mass of pilin used in the vaccine (5 mg per dose); earlier studies had only reported standardized amounts of pilin used in vaccines based on spectrophotometric measurements of percent light transmittance at specific wavelengths.

Further support for use of pilin as a vaccine antigen came from experimental vaccine-challenge studies on piliated and nonpiliated *M bovis* strain Epp 63.[32] In that study, calves administered two intramuscular doses, 28 days apart, of formalin-killed piliated *M bovis* Epp 63 cells adjuvanted with aluminum hydroxide (percentage not described) had significantly lower clinical lesion scores and significantly higher pilin-specific serum IgG titers versus control calves, and were considered protected against homologous *M bovis* challenge.

A pilin-based native pilin vaccine (two SC doses of 200 μg per dose, 21 days apart, adjuvanted with aluminum hydroxide plus oil) was evaluated for its ability to protect calves against homologous and heterologous challenge.[17] In that study serum and tear levels of IgG and tear IgA were measured using a pilin-specific ELISA. This study reported significant protection from homologous challenge following vaccination, and correlations between protection and lacrimal IgG and IgA; challenge seemed to elevate tear IgG and IgA levels against challenge strain pilin type.

Results from a subsequent study with a similar vaccine dose (200 μg pilin adjuvanted with aluminum hydroxide plus oil given as two SC doses, 21 days apart) reported evidence for cross-reacting antipilin serum antibody responses to shared pilin antigens across different pilus serogroups.[33] Further investigation into pilin-based vaccines demonstrated that low doses (30 μg in FIA administered twice SC, 21 days apart) of recombinant pilin could stimulate serum agglutinating antibody responses against whole *M bovis* that seemed to protect calves against experimental homologous challenge.[34]

A subsequent study evaluated the ability of a vaccine composed of homologous cloned pili plus native pili (in FIA) representing all seven pilin serogroups to protect calves against homologous and heterologous challenge with *M bovis*; vaccines were administered SC and boostered between 4 and 6 weeks following primary vaccination.[35] The study reported benefits from vaccination with multivalent pilin vaccines at protecting calves against *M bovis* challenge. It was noted that systemic *M bovis* agglutinating antibody responses were blunted in cattle receiving a multivalent pilin vaccine versus a monovalent pilin vaccine, presumably as a result of antigenic competition; however, vaccines were still considered to be protective. Another interesting observation from that study was the apparent switching of *M bovis* from one pilin serogroup to another, possibly in response to the presence of specific antibody in ocular tissues and fluids.

Mucosally Administered *Moraxella bovis* Pili

When native *M bovis* pili were adjuvanted with a series of different test adjuvants and administered intranasally (IN) to 6- to 8-month-old Angus beef calves, anti-*M bovis* pilin IgA responses in tears could be demonstrated with certain adjuvants.[36] The adjuvants that stimulated significantly higher tear antipilin IgA responses versus control calves given adjuvants alone were saponin from QuilA, and a mixture of mineral oil plus sorbitan monooleate plus polyoxyethylene sorbitan monooleate (Marcol Span). In that study, calves received IN vaccines in both nostrils (3 mL per nostril; total pilin dose per vaccination was 500 μg) on Days 0 and 15; tears were sampled on Days 0, 15, and then every 30 days through Day 135. Significantly higher (vs Day 0) antipilin IgA in tears were measured at Days 45, 75, 105, and 135 in calves administered pilin + QuilA and pilin + Marcol Span versus calves given QuilA and Marcol Span adjuvant alone. In this study the antipilin tear IgA responses did not seem to have any effect on *M bovis* isolations from eyes or the development of naturally occurring IBK in these calves. The method of tear collection used in this study (manual stimulation of the conjunctiva and tear collection with a dropper) may have led to variations in the tear volume produced between animals. For this reason, it is possible that standardization of tear samples using total sample IgA or total tear protein used in the ELISA assays may have improved the ability to correlate antipilin IgA responses with IBK development.

Cytotoxin (Hemolysin): Systemic Immune Response Following Naturally Occurring Infectious Bovine Keratoconjunctivitis and Experimental Moraxella bovis Infections

One of the initial reports characterizing the cytotoxin (hemolysin) of *M bovis* demonstrated at least two-fold increases in serum hemolysin neutralizing titers in seven of eight calves during development of clinical IBK.[37] Cattle with naturally occurring IBK were subsequently reported to develop antihemolysin serum antibodies over the 30-day period in which an outbreak of IBK occurred; serum titers to hemolysin were reported to last up to 7 years following IBK.[38] Other notable findings from this study were that antihemolysin activity cross-reacted with multiple *M bovis* isolates and that formalin treatment of purified *M bovis* membrane fractions destroyed antihemolytic antibody formation in vaccinated mice. A similar finding of an increase in the ability of serum to neutralize leukocidic and hemolytic activities of *M bovis* from calves between preinoculation to 10 to 38 days postinoculation was also reported.[39]

Parenterally Administered Moraxella bovis/Moraxella bovoculi Cytotoxin (Hemolysin)

A vaccine containing approximately 1 mg total protein that was enriched in hemolysin derived from nonpiliated *M bovis* cultures (two SC doses given 28 days apart; inactivated with 2% formalin and containing FIA) was reported to provide some protection in 4- to 6-month-old beef calves from heterologous *M bovis* challenge.[40] In this study, systemic, but not tear, hemolysis-inhibiting antibody titers were detected. Authors noted the importance of cross-protective immunity being demonstrated with the hemolysin antigen, something that had not been achieved with *M bovis* pili-based vaccines.

A SC administered recombinant *M bovis* cytotoxin subunit vaccine comprised of the recombinant carboxy terminus of *M bovis* cytotoxin (designated MbxA; 500 μg/vaccine dose) adjuvanted with immune-stimulating complex matrices (ISCOMs) was evaluated in a blinded randomized controlled field trial in 2- to 8-month-old beef calves.[41] Among the MbxA vaccinated calves, the Day 0 (prevaccination) to Week 7 (3 weeks postbooster) changes in cytotoxin-specific IgG in serum versus tears were directly correlated. Among the saline control calves in this study, the Day 0 to Day 42 mean change in MbxA-specific tear IgA ratios was more than twice as high in ulcerated (mean = 0.44; SE = 0.27; n = 12) versus nonulcerated (mean = 0.19; SE = 0.19; n = 17) saline control calves; however, these differences were not significant (P = .44) and minimal changes were observed in tear IgG ratios in the same subset of animals. A significant reduction in the proportion of calves with IBK was observed at Week 12 in the MbxA vaccinates (0.303) versus the saline (0.586) and adjuvant (0.516) control groups; however, Week 20 differences between groups were not significant. Although there seemed to be some benefit for this vaccine to reduce IBK and shorten healing times in vaccinated calves, a tendency for larger ulcers in vaccinates led authors to speculate that ocular IgG-mediated complement fixation might exacerbate corneal injury in IBK by attracting neutrophils into the eye. This seemed plausible considering a previous observation that hydroxyurea-induced immunosuppression of dairy calves in conjunction with experimental challenge with M bovis led to shallower but larger ulcers compared with control calves.[42]

To determine if additional protective antigens could enhance the ability of an M bovis cytotoxin vaccine to prevent naturally occurring IBK, a subsequent blinded randomized controlled field study was done in beef calves where the vaccine antigen was a recombinant fusion protein comprised of the amino-terminal conserved region of the seven M bovis serogroups along with the carboxy terminus of MbxA (pilin-MbxA) adjuvanted with ISCOM-matrices (500 µg protein per dose; two SC doses, 21 days apart).[43] Significantly higher median changes (Day 0–42 and Day 0–126) in M bovis cytotoxin serum neutralizing titers were observed in MbxA vaccinates versus adjuvant control calves. The Week 9 and Week 18 proportion of ulcerated calves were lower in pilin-MbxA vaccinates (0.24 and 0.35, respectively) compared with adjuvant control calves (0.33 and 0.46, respectively); however, these differences were not significant. In looking at the frequency of bacterial isolations from initial ulcers, M bovis was cultured more frequently in the initial ulcers of control calves (7 of 15 ulcers) versus MbxA (2 of 18 ulcers) or pilin-MbxA (4 of 12 ulcers) vaccinates. Additionally, M bovoculi was cultured more frequently from MbxA (14 of 18 ulcers) and pilin-MbxA (6 of 12 ulcers) vaccinates versus adjuvant control calves (7 of 15 ulcers). This study raised the possibility that the presence of M bovoculi in a herd could reduce efficacy of an M bovis vaccine against IBK.

The efficacy of a recombinant M bovoculi cytotoxin subunit vaccine adjuvanted with ISCOM matrices to prevent naturally occurring IBK was also evaluated in beef calves.[44] The vaccine contained 500 µg of recombinant M bovoculi cytotoxin (MbvA) and was given as a 2-mL dose SC and boostered 21 days later. In this study, Day 0 to 42 changes in M bovoculi cytotoxin neutralizing serum titers were significantly higher in vaccinates versus control calves; however, there was no difference in the cumulative proportions of ulcerated calves between groups.

In a subsequent vaccine efficacy study, recombinant M bovis pilin-cytotoxin plus recombinant M bovoculi cytotoxin were adjuvanted with ISCOM matrices and administered to beef calves (two SC doses, 21 days apart).[45] Significantly higher fold changes to M bovoculi serum cytotoxin neutralizing antibody titers in nonulcerated vaccinated calves could be demonstrated from Day 0 to Day 42 versus control calves that received adjuvant alone. However, changes in M bovis serum cytotoxin neutralizing titers in nonulcerated vaccinated calves versus control calves were not significantly different. Antibody responses to the pilin component of this vaccine were not evaluated. The proportions of calves that developed IBK between control and vaccine groups was not significantly different. This study concluded that additional antigens, novel adjuvants, and alternate routes of vaccine administration might improve the efficacy of recombinant subunit Moraxella spp vaccines against IBK.

Mucosally Administered Moraxella bovis Cytotoxin (Hemolysin)

MbxA adjuvanted with polyacrylic acid, a mucoadhesive polymer, was evaluated for its ability to stimulate mucosal antibody responses in 11- to 13-month-old beef steers following IN vaccination.[46] Low (200 µg) and high (500 µg) vaccine doses of MbxA were included in the 2-mL vaccines (administered as 1 mL per nostril) on Days 0 and 21; control steers received adjuvant alone. Significant differences were observed between vaccine and control groups in the change in tear IgA ratios (a calculated value that took into account the protein concentration of each tear sample) between Day 0 (day of primary vaccine dose) and Days 28, 42, and 55, with the highest changes occurring in the two cytotoxin-vaccinated groups; however, post hoc comparison between groups were not significantly different. No significant differences were observed between groups in changes from Day 0 to Days 28, 42, or 55 in tear cytotoxin-specific tear IgG, or serum or tear cytotoxin neutralizing titer. A subsequent study in beef steers compared partially solubilized versus precipitated (particulate) formulations of MbxA (500 μg) adjuvanted with polyacrylic acid.[47] Dosing was performed as in the earlier study, except that the booster was given on Day 28. This study reported significantly higher fold changes in MbxA-specific IgG in serum and tear samples and MbxA-neutralizing antibody titers in tears from steers that received the particulate formulation.[47]

Results from these studies suggest that IN vaccination may hold promise for stimulating mucosal antibody responses to *Moraxella* spp antigens in cattle; however, there remains a lack of information regarding what constitutes a protective immune response against IBK. Therefore, future predictions as to the potential for success of IN vaccines to prevent IBK remains speculative.

EVIDENCE FOR PROTECTIVE IMMUNE RESPONSES TO *MORAXELLA* ANTIGENS

Results of experimental research conducted over the past 50 years has provided glimpses into what types of immune responses might protect against IBK associated with *Moraxella* spp infections; however, challenges exist in interpreting results from investigations where different types of immune responses were measured and different *Moraxella* spp antigens were used to quantitate systemic versus mucosal responses.

A survey of Nigerian cattle reported higher serum hemagglutinating antibody (HA) titers in unaffected Zebu cattle compared with affected Friesian cattle; the antibody assay used in this study incorporated a noncellular supernatant fraction derived from whole *M bovis* as antigen.[48] The higher titers supported a possible role for serum antibodies in protection against IBK.

Early studies into mucosal immune responses to ocular infections with *M bovis* suggested that enhanced local ocular defense mechanisms accounted for the observed resistance of 4- to 6-month-old beef and dairy calves to *M bovis* re-exposure in an ocular irradiation model of IBK.[49] Further investigation into these local defense mechanisms found that IgA specific for *M bovis* antigens was a major component of ocular secretions in calves that had severe IBK.[10] These authors concluded that there was a need for further studies to identify which antigens of *M bovis* are responsible for protective immunity and for studies into local administration of *M bovis* vaccines, bacterins, or antigens.

When an intrathird eyelid injection of an autogenous *M bovis* bacterin (vaccine details not provided by authors) was evaluated, protection against establishment of hemolytic *M bovis* or development of IBK were deemed to be limited despite reduced rates of hemolytic *M bovis* isolations and clinical IBK from eyes of vaccinates versus nonvaccinates.[50] When this same research group evaluated tears for the presence of HA directed at a formalized and sonicated whole *M bovis* antigen, it was determined that intrathird eyelid vaccination of an autogenous *M bovis* bacterin did not result in increased HA tear titers; however, there seemed to be an inverse relationship between HA titer and *M bovis* isolation from study calves in that the percent of calves with *M bovis* isolations decreased with increasing mean HA titer.[51]

When *M bovis*–specific IgM, IgG, and secretory IgA was quantified in a closed herd of beef calves that was naturally affected with IBK over the course of one summer, it was reported that the highest titer-specific antibody in lacrimal secretions to *M bovis* was IgG, whereas secretory IgA was generally lowest.[52] The possibility that calves were not protected from IBK because of a lack of *M bovis*–specific IgA was considered, and suggests that mucosal vaccination routes might be advantageous for boosting secretory IgA levels in tear fluid.

In 3- to 4-month-old dairy calves infected with *M bovis* using an irradiation model of infection, positive associations were identified between the presence of *M bovis*–specific lacrimal antibodies, improvement of clinical IBK, and decreased numbers of *M bovis* that could be isolated from conjunctival swabs.[53] In this study tear antibody measurements were made using a passive hemagglutination test with tannic acid–treated sheep red blood cells that were sensitized with a whole *M bovis* cell sonicate.

In experimental vaccination-challenge studies, cattle vaccinated parenterally with *M bovis* pili or piliated strains of *M bovis* seem to have some protection against homologous *M bovis* challenge. Although the presence of pilin-specific IgG and IgA in tears seemed to correlate with protection in one study,[17] a more recent study could not conclusively demonstrate a beneficial role for antipilin tear IgA in conferring resistance to IBK.[36] Studies demonstrating cross-neutralizing ability of antihemolysin antibodies suggest that antibody responses to cytotoxin have the capacity to neutralize cytotoxins from diverse *M bovis* strains.[38]

In one limited study of calves (two 3-month-old Hereford calves and two 4- to 6-week-old Holstein calves) that were experimentally challenged with *M bovis*, calves that resisted challenge re-exposures to *M bovis* 6 months following induction of acute IBK were noted to have lacrimal whole *M bovis* cell-specific IgA as measured with an ELISA; authors concluded that specific IgA antibodies in tear secretions could be used as a reliable indicator of *M bovis*–induced IBK resistance and suggested that vaccine development should focus on methods to augment specific IgA antibodies in tear secretions.[54]

EVIDENCE FOR HARMFUL IMMUNE RESPONSES TO *MORAXELLA* ANTIGENS

During experimental ocular *M bovis* infections of dairy calves that were neutrophil depleted with hydroxyurea, corneal ulcers caused by *M bovis* were observed to be larger but more shallow compared with nonhydroxyurea-treated control calves.[42] Calves that were vaccinated with recombinant *M bovis* cytotoxin formulations were observed to have larger corneal ulcers at initial diagnosis, although the differences versus control calves were not statistically significant.[41,43] Given that tear IgG is derived from plasma and that this transfer is increased during the development of keratoconjunctivitis,[55] the possibility exists that systemic IgG to *Moraxella* spp antigens could exacerbate corneal injury following *Moraxella* spp antigen-antibody binding in the eye leading to complement fixation, release of complement factors, and subsequent attraction of neutrophils into ocular tissues. Release of degradative enzymes from neutrophils lysed by cytotoxins of *Moraxella* spp might worsen corneal injury in IBK. Because IgA does not fix complement, mucosal vaccination methods that stimulate ocular IgA against *Moraxella* spp antigens could offer advantages over parenterally administered *Moraxella* spp vaccines.

SUMMARY

Over the past 50 years numerous studies have been conducted to discover more effective vaccines to prevent IBK. Although most studies have focused on parenterally administered vaccines, more recent studies have begun to investigate mucosal vaccines. Most studies have focused on whole-cell *M bovis* bacterins (in some cases these are piliated), native or recombinant pili, hemolytic/cytolytic-enriched fractions derived from *Moraxella* spp cultures, or recombinant *M bovis/M bovoculi* cytotoxin. However, critical knowledge gaps remain in regard to which *Moraxella* spp antigens alone or in combination are protective, and whether systemic, mucosal, or both types of immune responses are more important in protecting cattle against IBK associated with *Moraxella* spp. A variety of other cellular constituents from *M bovis* and *M bovoculi* exist, and whole genome sequencing of both organisms has opened up new avenues for investigating such factors. Recent evidence that *Moraxella* spp are opportunistic pathogens residing as commensals in the URT and eye raises further questions regarding possible imprinting of systemic and mucosal immune responses. Further studies are required to determine if commensal *Moraxella* spp induce immune regulatory responses that limit vaccine immunogenicity and efficacy. Novel vaccine antigens, formulations, or delivery vehicles may be required to circumvent immune regulatory responses and induce antibody or T-cell responses of sufficient magnitude and duration to prevent IBK.

CLINICS CARE POINTS

- In experimental vaccine studies, *Moraxella bovis* and *Moraxella bovoculi* can stimulate systemic and local immune responses in cattle.

- More recent randomized controlled field studies have not demonstrated benefit from some parenterally administered commercially available or autogenous *Moraxella* spp. bacterins.

- In some experimental vaccine studies, vaccination of pregnant cows prior to parturition provided some protection against IBK in calves.

DISCLOSURE

The authors have nothing to disclose.

REFERENCES

1. Knop E, Knop N. Anatomy and immunology of the ocular surface. Chem Immunol Allergy 2007;92:36–49.
2. Lima SF, Teixeira AG, Higgins CH, et al. The upper respiratory tract microbiome and its potential role in bovine respiratory disease and otitis media. Sci Rep 2016; 6:29050.
3. Cullen JN, Lithio A, Seetharam AS, et al. Microbial community sequencing analysis of the calf eye microbiota and relationship to infectious bovine keratoconjunctivitis. Vet Microbiol 2017;207:267–79.
4. Menaka R, Puri G. Role of lacrimal gland in tear production in different animal species: a review. Livestock Research International 2015;3(2):40–2.
5. Eidet JR, Dartt DA, Utheim TP. Concise review: comparison of culture membranes used for tissue engineered conjunctival epithelial equivalents. J Funct Biomater 2015;6(4):1064–84.
6. Hoorens PR, Rinaldi M, Li RW, et al. Genome wide analysis of the bovine mucin genes and their gastrointestinal transcription profile. BMC Genomics 2011; 12:140.

7. Pinard CL, Weiss ML, Brightman AH, et al. Normal anatomical and histochemical characteristics of the lacrimal glands in the American bison and cattle. Anat Histol Embryol 2003;32(5):257–62.

8. Knop E, Knop N. The role of eye-associated lymphoid tissue in corneal immune protection. J Anat 2005;206(3):271–85.

9. Mach JP, Pahud JJ. Secretory IgA, a major immunoglobulin in most bovine external secretions. J Immunol 1971;106(2):552–63.

10. Nayar PS, Saunders JR. Infectious bovine keratoconjunctivitis II. Antibodies in lacrimal secretions of cattle naturally or experimentally infected with Moraxella bovis. Can J Comp Med 1975;39(1):32–40.

11. Bayraktaroğlu AG, Aştı RN. Light and electron microscopic studies on Conjunctiva Associated Lymphoid Tissue (CALT) in cattle. Revue de médecine vétérinaire 2009;160(5):252–7.

12. Mirabzadeh-Ardakani A, Solie J, Gonzalez-Cano P, et al. Tissue- and age-dependent expression of the bovine DEFB103 gene and protein. Cell Tissue Res 2016;363(2):479–90.

13. Roussey JA, Oliveira LJ, Langohr IM, et al. Regulatory T cells and immune profiling in Johne's disease lesions. Vet Immunol Immunopathol 2016;181:39–50.

14. Osman R, Malmuthuge N, Gonzalez-Cano P, et al. Development and function of the mucosal immune system in the upper respiratory tract of neonatal calves. Annu Rev Anim Biosci 2018;6:141–55.

15. Midla LT, Hill K, Van Engen NK, et al. Innate and acquired immune responses following intranasal vaccination with two commercially available modified-live viral vaccines in colostrum fed neonatal Holstein calves. J Am Vet Med Assoc, in press.

16. Gould S, Dewell R, Tofflemire K, et al. Randomized blinded challenge study to assess association between Moraxella bovoculi and Infectious Bovine Keratoconjunctivitis in dairy calves. Vet Microbiol 2013;164(1–2):108–15.

17. Lepper AW. Vaccination against infectious bovine keratoconjunctivitis: protective efficacy and antibody response induced by pili of homologous and heterologous strains of Moraxella bovis. Aust Vet J 1988;65(10):310–6.

18. Griffin JF. A strategic approach to vaccine development: animal models, monitoring vaccine efficacy, formulation and delivery. Adv Drug Deliv Rev 2002;54(6):851–61.

19. Hughes DE, Pugh GW Jr. Experimentally induced bovine infectious keratoconjunctivitis: effectiveness of intramuscular vaccination with viable Moraxella bovis culture. Am J Vet Res 1971;32(6):879–86.

20. Hughes DE, Pugh GW Jr. Experimentally induced infectious bovine keratoconjunctivitis: vaccination with nonviable Moraxella bovis culture. Am J Vet Res 1972;33(12):2475–9.

21. Pugh GW Jr, Hughes DE, Schulz VD, et al. Experimentally induced infectious bovine keratoconjunctivitis: resistance of vaccinated cattle to homologous and heterologous strains of Moraxella bovis. Am J Vet Res 1976;37(1):57–60.

22. Pugh GW Jr, McDonald TJ, Kopecky KE. Experimental infectious bovine keratoconjunctivitis: efficacy of a vaccine prepared from nonhemolytic strains of Moraxella bovis. Am J Vet Res 1982;43(6):1081–4.

23. Bishop B, Schurig GG, Troutt HF. Enzyme-linked immunosorbent assay for measurement of anti-Moraxella bovis antibodies. Am J Vet Res 1982;43(8):1443–5.

24. Gerber JD, Selzer NL, Sharpee RL, et al. Immunogenicity of a Moraxella bovis bacterin containing attachment and cornea-degrading enzyme antigens. Vet Immunol Immunopathol 1988;18(1):41–52.

25. Gerber JD, Inventor. *Moraxella bovis* Protease Vaccine; US Patent No. 4,675,176. June 23, 1987.

26. Misiura M. Keratoconjunctivitis infections in calves: attempt at elimination by active immunization. Arch Vet Pol 1994;34(3–4):187–94.

27. Misiura M. Estimation of fimbrial vaccine effectiveness in protection against keratoconjunctivitis infections in calves considering different routes of introducing vaccine antigene. Arch Vet Pol 1994;34(3–4):177–86.

28. Pugh GW Jr, Hughes DE, Booth GD. Experimentally induced infections bovine keratoconjunctivitis: effectiveness of a pilus vaccine against exposure to homologous strains of *Moraxella bovis*. Am J Vet Res 1977;38(10):1519–22.

29. Pugh GW Jr, Kopecky KE, McDonald TJ. Infectious bovine keratoconjunctivitis: enhancement of *Moraxella bovis* pili immunogenicity with diphtheria-tetanus toxoids and pertussis vaccine. Am J Vet Res 1984;45(4):661–5.

30. Pugh GW Jr, Kopecky KE, McDonald TJ. Infectious bovine keratoconjunctivitis: subconjunctival administration of a *Moraxella bovis* pilus preparation enhances immunogenicity. Am J Vet Res 1985;46(4):811–5.

31. Lehr C, Jayappa HG, Goodnow RA. Serologic and protective characterization of *Moraxella bovis* pili. Cornell Vet 1985;75(4):484–92.

32. Jayappa HG, Lehr C. Pathogenicity and immunogenicity of piliated and nonpiliated phases of *Moraxella bovis* in calves. Am J Vet Res 1986;47(10):2217–21.

33. Lepper AW, Moore LJ, Atwell JL, et al. The protective efficacy of pili from different strains of *Moraxella bovis* within the same serogroup against infectious bovine keratoconjunctivitis. Vet Microbiol 1992;32(2):177–87.

34. Lepper AW, Elleman TC, Hoyne PA, et al. A *Moraxella bovis* pili vaccine produced by recombinant DNA technology for the prevention of infectious bovine keratoconjunctivitis. Vet Microbiol 1993;36(1–2):175–83.

35. Lepper AW, Atwell JL, Lehrbach PR, et al. The protective efficacy of cloned *Moraxella bovis* pili in monovalent and multivalent vaccine formulations against experimentally induced infectious bovine keratoconjunctivitis (IBK). Vet Microbiol 1995;45(2–3):129–38.

36. Zbrun MV, Zielinski GC, Piscitelli HC, et al. Evaluation of anti-*Moraxella bovis* pili immunoglobulin-A in tears following intranasal vaccination of cattle. Res Vet Sci 2012;93(1):183–9.

37. Nakazawa M, Nemoto H. Hemolytic activity of *Moraxella bovis*. Nippon Juigaku Zasshi 1979;41(4):363–7.

38. Ostle AG, Rosenbusch RF. Immunogenicity of *Moraxella bovis* hemolysin. Am J Vet Res 1985;46(5):1011–4.

39. Hoien-Dalen PS, Rosenbusch RF, Roth JA. Comparative characterization of the leukocidic and hemolytic activity of *Moraxella bovis*. Am J Vet Res 1990;51(2):191–6.

40. Billson FM, Hodgson JL, Egerton JR, et al. A haemolytic cell-free preparation of *Moraxella bovis* confers protection against infectious bovine keratoconjunctivitis. FEMS Microbiol Lett 1994;124(1):69–74.

41. Angelos JA, Hess JF, George LW. Prevention of naturally occurring infectious bovine keratoconjunctivitis with a recombinant *Moraxella bovis* cytotoxin-ISCOM matrix adjuvanted vaccine. Vaccine 2004;23(4):537–45.

42. Kagonyera GM, George LW, Munn R. Light and electron microscopic changes in corneas of healthy and immunomodulated calves infected with *Moraxella bovis*. Am J Vet Res 1988;49(3):386–95.

43. Angelos JA, Bonifacio RG, Ball LM, et al. Prevention of naturally occurring infectious bovine keratoconjunctivitis with a recombinant *Moraxella bovis* pilin-

Moraxella bovis cytotoxin-ISCOM matrix adjuvanted vaccine. Vet Microbiol 2007; 125(3–4):274–83.

44. Angelos JA, Lane VM, Ball LM, et al. Recombinant *Moraxella bovoculi* cytotoxin-ISCOM matrix adjuvanted vaccine to prevent naturally occurring infectious bovine keratoconjunctivitis. Vet Res Commun 2010;34(3):229–39.

45. Angelos JA, Gohary KG, Ball LM, et al. Randomized controlled field trial to assess efficacy of a *Moraxella bovis* pilin-cytotoxin-*Moraxella bovoculi* cytotoxin subunit vaccine to prevent naturally occurring infectious bovine keratoconjunctivitis. Am J Vet Res 2012;73(10):1670–5.

46. Angelos JA, Edman JM, Chigerwe M. Ocular immune responses in steers following intranasal vaccination with recombinant *Moraxella bovis* cytotoxin adjuvanted with polyacrylic acid. Clin Vaccine Immunol 2014;21(2):181–7.

47. Angelos JA, Chigerwe M, Edman JM, et al. Systemic and ocular immune responses in cattle following intranasal vaccination with precipitated or partially solubilized recombinant *Moraxella bovis* cytotoxin adjuvanted with polyacrylic acid. Am J Vet Res 2016;77(12):1411–8.

48. Makinde AA, Ezeh AO, Onoviran O, et al. Prevalence of serum antibodies to *Moraxella bovis* in cattle in Nigeria. Br Vet J 1985;141(6):643–6.

49. Nayar PS, Saunders JR. Infectious bovine keratoconjunctivitis I. Experimental production. Can J Comp Med 1975;39(1):22–31.

50. Arora AK, Killinger AH, Mansfield ME. Bacteriologic and vaccination studies in a field epizootic of infectious bovine keratoconjunctivitis in calves. Am J Vet Res 1976;37(7):803–5.

51. Arora AK, Killinger AH, Myers WL. Detection of *Moraxella bovis* antibodies in infectious bovine keratoconjunctivitis by a passive hemagglutination test. Am J Vet Res 1976;37(12):1489–92.

52. Killinger AH, Weisiger RM, Helper LC, et al. Detection of *Moraxella bovis* antibodies in the SIgA, IgG, and IgM classes of immunoglobulin in bovine lacrimal secretions by an indirect fluorescent antibody test. Am J Vet Res 1978;39(6): 931–4.

53. Weech GM, Renshaw HW. Infectious bovine keratoconjunctivitis: bacteriologic, immunologic, and clinical responses of cattle to experimental exposure with *Moraxella bovis*. Comp Immunol Microbiol Infect Dis 1983;6(1):81–94.

54. Smith PC, Greene WH, Allen JW. Antibodies related to resistance in bovine pinkeye. California Veterinarian 1989;43(4):7–10.

55. Pedersen KB. The origin of immunoglobulin-G in bovine tears. Acta Pathol Microbiol Scand B Microbiol Immunol 1973;81(2):245–52.

Applying Concepts of Causal Inference to Infectious Bovine Keratoconjunctivitis

Annette M. O'Connor, BVSc, MVSc, DVSc, FANZCVS

KEYWORDS

- Bradford Hill viewpoints • Causal inference • Infectious bovine keratoconjunctivitis
- *Moraxella* • Study design

KEY POINTS

- The assessment of causation requires evaluation of different forms of evidence.
- Based on Bradford Hill viewpoints there is evidence to support a causal role for *Moraxella bovis* in infectious bovine keratoconjunctivitis.
- Most of the evidence base for *Moraxella bovis* comes from laboratory and experimental evidence.
- Based on Bradford Hill viewpoints there is little evidence to support a causal role for *Moraxella bovoculi* in infectious bovine keratoconjunctivitis.

INTRODUCTION

This article discusses the application of causal assessment frameworks to understanding putative infectious causes of infectious bovine keratoconjunctivitis (IBK), that is, *Moraxella bovis* and *Moraxella bovoculi*.

CAUSAL FRAMEWORKS

Establishing causation, otherwise known as causal assessment, is a difficult task. A task made more difficult by the variety of causal assessment frameworks available to consider. There are currently two frameworks for establishing causation that seem to dominate in the veterinary sciences: Koch postulates (or the Henle-Koch postulates) and the Bradford Hill viewpoints.

Koch's postulates are based on three criteria[1]:

- The parasite occurs in every case of the disease in question and under circumstances that can account for the pathologic changes and clinical course of the disease.

The author has nothing to disclose.
Department of Large Animal Clinical Sciences, College of Veterinary Medicine, Michigan State University, 784 Wilson Road, Room G-100, East Lansing, MI 48824, USA
E-mail address: Oconn445@msu.edu

- It occurs in no other disease as a fortuitous and nonpathogenic parasite.
- After being fully isolated from the body and repeatedly grown in pure culture, it can induce the disease anew.

The issue with Koch postulates in microbiology is that ready examples that need exceptions are easy to identify: virology, asymptomatic infections, microbiome, commensal bacteria, and biofilms.[1,2] Therefore as a generalizable framework, Koch postulates are often found wanting.

Bradford Hill viewpoints (occasionally and incorrectly called causal criteria) are more extensive and broadly applicable.[3] Bradford Hill viewpoints were initially developed to aid in concluding that lung cancer was caused by smoking. Since initially proposed, Bradford Hill viewpoints have been used for many outcomes and putative causes. The advantage of the viewpoints is that they can be applied to outcomes beyond disease and still have utility. For example, the viewpoints can assess causes of such diseases as diabetes, lung cancer, and AIDS. Yet, the viewpoints can also be used in nondisease outcomes of interest, such as low grades for students and recidivism. As such, one of the reasons for the durability of Bradford Hill viewpoints is perhaps the unique advantage over Koch of applying to any causal factor or outcome: microbiological, social, societal, behavioral, environmental, genetic, or nutritional. The viewpoints are as follows:

1. Strength (effect size): A small association does not mean that there is not a causal effect, although the larger the association, the more likely that it is causal.
2. Consistency (reproducibility): Consistent findings observed by different persons in different places with different samples strengthens the likelihood of an effect.
3. Specificity: Causation is likely if there is a specific population at a specific site and disease with no other likely explanation. The more specific an association between a factor and an effect is, the bigger the probability of a causal relationship.
4. Temporality: The effect has to occur after the cause (and if there is an expected delay between the cause and expected effect, then the effect must occur after that delay).
5. Biologic gradient (dose–response relationship): Greater exposure should generally lead to greater incidence of the effect. However, in some cases, the mere presence of the factor can trigger the effect. In other cases, an inverse proportion is observed: greater exposure leads to lower incidence.
6. Plausibility: A plausible mechanism between cause and effect is helpful (but Hill noted that knowledge of the mechanism is limited by current knowledge).
7. Coherence: Coherence between epidemiologic and laboratory findings increases the likelihood of an effect. However, Hill noted that "... lack of such [laboratory] evidence cannot nullify the epidemiologic effect on associations."
8. Experiment: Occasionally it is possible to appeal to experimental evidence.
9. Analogy: The use of analogies or similarities between the observed association and any other associations.

Some authors also consider reversibility: if the cause is deleted then the effect should disappear. However, this concept can be captured by experimental evidence. The approach to applying Bradford Hill viewpoints should be considered as a building of evidence. The more viewpoints that a putative causal factor has in association with the outcome, the greater the evidence base for a causal relationship. The viewpoint list is not a checklist and should not be treated as such. Failure to have one or several factors is not proof against causation, just as having one or several viewpoints are not proof of causation. The viewpoints have, however, stood the test of time since first proposed. An example of the recent applications of the viewpoints for causal assessment is the 2015 outbreak of microcephaly in South America, which was rapidly and unexpectedly associated with Zika virus.[4] Zika virus has been known for many years and associated with a mild, self-limiting disease until an outbreak of microcephaly in South America in 2015 was associated with Zika virus infection. Subsequent evaluation of Bradford Hill viewpoints by several groups illustrated the viewpoints' utility and suggested that the relationship was causal.[5–7] Note that Rasmussen and coworkers[7] also reviewed the evidence for Zika being a cause of microcephaly, a set of seven criteria for "proof" of human teratogenicity proposed by Shepard.[8] In this discussion about causation for IBK, Bradford Hill viewpoints for causal assessment are used. Readers interested in other frameworks for assessing causation and those generally interested in understanding causal frameworks better are directed to other sources.[9–11]

BRADFORD HILL VIEWPOINTS APPLIED TO *MORAXELLA BOVIS, MORAXELLA BOVOCULI,* AND INFECTIOUS BOVINE KERATOCONJUNCTIVITIS

In the following sections Bradford Hill viewpoints are applied to the two infectious pathogens most frequently associated with IBK, and how the viewpoints can be applied to assess the causal relationship is discussed.

Strength (Effect Size)

A small association does not mean that there is not a causal effect, although the larger the association, the more likely that it is causal. This viewpoint is generally considered to refer to comparisons of results from observational studies. The effect size measures the strength of an association. The term "effect size" refers to a metric that compares disease incidence in the exposed with disease incidence in the unexposed, assuming all confounding factors are controlled.

The effect size metric is measured in several ways, depending on the study design. For a pathogen like *M bovis*, the effect size metric would usually be incidence risk ratio, incidence rate ratio, or incidence odds ratio. The risk ratio comes from the comparison of the incidence risk of IBK in animals exposed to the putative risk factor for a defined period (*M bovis, M bovoculi*) compared with the incidence risk of IBK in animals not exposed to the putative risk factor in the same defined period. Incidence risk is the number of new cases divided by the number unexposed. The ratio of these two proportions, rather than the difference, is usually used for mathematical reasons.

Another possible effect size metric is the rate ratio. The rate ratio is obtained from a comparison of the rate of new cases of IBK in animals exposed to the putative risk factor (eg, *M bovis* or *M bovoculi*) divided by the rate of new cases of IBK in animals exposed to the putative risk factor of interest. Rate is given by the number of new rates divided by the time at risk.

The incidence odds ratio is another effect size metric. The incidence odds in the exposed is given by the number of new cases of IBK divided by the number of noncases of IBK in the exposed. The incidence odds in the unexposed is given by the number of new cases of IBK divided by the number of noncases of IBK in the unexposed. The incidence odds ratio is simply the ratio of those odds. Researchers can obtain the incidence risk ratio, incidence rate ratio, or incidence odds ratio directly by conducting a cohort study or indirectly by conducting an incidence case-control design.

Using the risk ratio and *M bovis* as an example, the ideal approach to generating this type of evidence would be to conduct a population-based cohort study by enrolling IBK-free calves, determining if they are *M bovis*–negative and *M bovis*–

positive, and then follow the calves over time. At the end of the study period, the investigator would calculate the incidence risk ratio by dividing the risk of IBK in the *M bovis* calves by the risk of IBK in the *M bovis*–negative calves. If the risk of IBK were greater in the calves with *M bovis* compared with those without *M bovis*, then the incidence risk ratio would be greater than one; if there were no difference in risk, then the incidence risk ratio would be close to one; and if the incidence risk ratio was less than one, this would imply being infected with *M bovis* protected against IBK.

Surprisingly, there is a dearth of cohort studies or incidence case-control that explicitly compare the incidence risk, incidence rate, or incidence odds of IBK for putative risk factors. One study conducted using this approach reported an adjusted hazard ratio (incidence risk ratio) for *M bovis* and IBK was 1.60 (95% confidence interval [CI], 0.48–5.53; *P* value = .44; n = 77). This is a modest effect size, with a wide level of confidence that incorporated certainty and did not suggest a strong association. For *M bovoculi*, the same study reported the adjusted hazard ratio (an incidence risk ratio) for *M bovoculi* was 1.38 (95% CI, 0.54–3.53; *P* = .49). As with *M bovis*, this a modest effect size only slightly closer to one than *M bovis*, with a wide level of confidence that did not suggest a strong association.[12] One study from Australia followed 20 calves with repeated samplings over 18 months, but this study did not directly compare isolation of *M bovis* in IBK cases compared with non-IBK cases.[13]

Other approaches to estimating an effect size would be to conduct a prevalence case-control study or cross-sectional study. Using *M bovis* as an example, a prevalence case-control design would sample calves with prevalent cases of IBK and calves without prevalence cases of IBK and compare the presence of *M bovis* in cases with control subjects. The cross-sectional design would sample a population of calves independent of IBK or *M bovis* status and then categorize the study subjects as having IBK or not and *M bovis*–positive or not. The major problem with such designs is the inference that the recovery of an organism obtained from an IBK lesion is equated with causation. In feedlot production, reaching conclusions about the causal organism based on culture results in lungs postmortem is problematic. It is unclear how problematic the concern is for IBK.

There are a few examples of prevalence comparison designs in the literature. In one such study, the effect size for *M bovis* and IBK is not reported, although it is reported that *M bovis* was more common in calves with IBK compared with calves without IBK.[14] In the study conducted by O'Connor and coworkers,[12] the adjusted prevalence ratio for *M bovoculi* in IBK lesions was 6.45 (95% CI, 3.35–12.44; *P* < .001), and the adjusted prevalence for *M bovis* in IBK lesions was 2.33 (95% CI, 1.22–4.45; *P* = .01).[12] This study clearly showed that *M bovoculi* was common in IBK lesions. Still, in the same group of cattle, IBK incidence was not associated with IBK (the incidence risk ratio was *M bovoculi*: 1.38 (95% CI, 0.54–3.53; *P* = .49).

It is theoretically possible to use the prevalence ratio from a cross-sectional or the prevalence odds ratio from a case-control study to estimate the incidence risk ratio or incidence odds ratio, respectively.[15] One of the critical assumptions required are that the prevalence of the exposure of interest (either *M bovis* or *M bovoculi*) is stable, that is, no change in prevalence from before to after the lesions occur, given the potential for secondary invasion of organisms into a purulent cornea.

Perhaps the most common observational study design is limited to IBK lesions and the prevalence of *M bovis* or *M bovoculi* in IBK lesions. This design is often based on diagnostic laboratory data, an accessible source of data. An example of such a design is a large retrospective study of IBK diagnostic cases submitted to the Nebraska

Veterinary Diagnostic Center (Lincoln, Nebraska) from July 1, 2010, through October 31, 2013. It is assumed the samples all came from IBK lesions, although this is not explicitly stated. A total of 1042 *Moraxella* isolates from 1538 swabs of lacrimal secretions collected from 282 herds from 30 US states were used in the study. *Moraxella* isolates were identified to the species level and were composed of *M bovoculi* (701 isolates), *M bovis* (295 isolates), *M ovis* (five isolates), and other *Moraxella* spp.[16] This result could suggest that *M bovoculi* is a more successful secondary invader of IBK lesions, that *M bovoculi* is easier to culture than *M bovis*, or that *M bovoculi* is a more common cause of IBK. However, based on the design, it is not possible to differentiate these options.

All of the previously mentioned studies attempted to assess causation at the individual level. Another approach is ecological. An ecological study assesses an association between more *M bovis* and *M bovoculi* and more incident IBK at the herd level. One study that used this approach evaluated *M bovis* and IBK over 5 years. The risk of IBK cases and *M bovis* were reported; there did seem to be an association between increases in isolation of hemolytic *M bovis* and new cases of IBK.[17] The data are reported in figures, and calculation of the correlation between organism isolation and new cases of IBK was not performed. Another study evaluated four herds each at one state of IBK: pre-IBK (n = 1 herd), acute IBK (n = 1 herd), post-IBK (n = 1 herd), and control (n = 1 herd). The study reported higher *M bovoculi* prevalence in conjunctival swabs in the pre-IBK and acute IBK compared with post-IBK and control herds and inferred.[18] The authors acknowledge this design's limitation for causal inference, that is, herd disease status is confounded by all other herd characteristics. However, the authors cautiously proposed that the results suggest that *M bovoculi* may be a cause of IBK because a high prevalence of *M bovoculi* in the pre-IBK herd and the acute IBK was found. The inference was that finding a high prevalence of IBK in the pre-IBK herd might refute the concept that *M bovoculi* is a secondary invader of lesions. Such an ecological approach is intriguing and should be pursued. However, ecological studies are susceptible to the ecological fallacy and do not provide direct evidence of causation at the individual level. Even if the high prevalence of *M bovoculi* is correlated with a high incidence of IBK, it will not be clear that *M bovoculi*–positive calves are the calves developing IBK. However, combined with other evidence at the individual level, such evidence could add to causal inference for either organism. Overall, this viewpoint is not met for either individual or herd-level studies.

Consistency (Reproducibility)

Consistent findings observed by different persons in different places with different samples strengthens the likelihood of an effect. The concept of consistency refers to observing the same association across multiple populations. This can refer to observational studies or clinical trials. For example, for smoking, the association between lung cancer and smoking is observed in multiple populations.[3] Lack of consistency was a major barrier for establishing that the Zika virus was a cause of microcephaly. Zika virus infection had, for many years, been considered a self-limiting disease, and therefore the association with microcephaly was inconsistent with previous studies. Frank and coworkers[6] reported: "no reports of adverse pregnancy or birth outcomes were noted during previous outbreaks of Zika virus disease in the Pacific Islands." However, over time the evidence seemed to increase, and multiple studies in multiple areas found an observational association of Zika with microcephaly and other congenital lesions.[4–7] It is worth noting that the evidence for consistency accumulated quickly for Zika and congenital microcephaly. This increase in evidence was likely caused by the researcher's community awareness that such information was needed for establishing causation.

For IBK, although it is true that multiple counties have reported that *M bovoculi* and *M bovis* are frequently isolated from ocular swabs of IBK lesions, such designs do not directly support causation. Too few studies are available that directly assess the incidence of IBK for either *M bovis* or *M bovoculi* to conclude that the associations are consistent. This viewpoint is not met for either individual or herd-level studies.

Specificity

Causation is likely if there is a very specific population at a specific site and disease with no other likely explanation. The more specific an association between a factor and an effect is, the bigger the probability of a causal relationship.

This viewpoint is usually not considered important to establishing causation, because many causes of disease are not specific. For example, smoking causes many cancers, not just lung cancer, but this lack of specificity does diminish the causal role of smoking in lung cancer. *M bovis* or *M bovoculi* do not seem to have an association with other diseases, although recently *Moraxella* were found to be more abundant in feedlot calves arriving with bovine respiratory disease.[19] This viewpoint is not met for either individual or herd-level studies.

Temporality

The effect has to occur after the cause (and if there is an expected delay between the cause and expected effect, then the effect must occur after that delay). This viewpoint aims to show that the incidence of IBK is higher in animals exposed to *M bovis* or *M bovoculi* compared with the incidence of IBK in animals not exposed to IBK, that is, the risk ratio or the rate ratio. Incidence could be measured as either a risk or a rate. To establish this viewpoint, it would be necessary to sample calves before disease occurrence and follow over time. The challenge with this design for the researcher is to know when such sampling should take place to ensure that the *M bovis* "status" of the eye is accurately captured. Furthermore, because IBK is an unpredictable disease, many calves would need to be sampled continuously (daily or weekly) in the hope that IBK occurs on the farm. One study has been conducted with this design approach and an incident outcome.[12] The study sampled randomly selected eye's and recorded subsequent incidence of IBK over a 3- to 6-week period. The study has four such periods for two different groups of calves from the same farm. Using a polymerase chain reaction–based detection method to detect *M bovis* in the eye swab and IBK incidence, the associations reported did not provide strong evidence to support the role of *M bovis* in IBK incidence. The adjusted hazard ratio for *M bovis* and IBK was 1.60 (95% CI, 0.48–5.53; $P = .44$; n = 77). This effect size estimate is positive, that is, the hazard of IBK was higher in calves with IBK detected before IBK occurrence. However, the uncertainty level is very high, with the 95% CI spanning an interval from 0.48 to 5.5. We are unaware of other studies that have used measured *M bovis* status before measuring IBK incidence. As mentioned in the strength of association viewpoint, many observational studies have evaluated the prevalence of *M bovis* in IBK lesions compared with *M bovis* in normal eyes, using a prevalent case-control design or cross-sectional design. However, such designs do not address the temporality viewpoint, and concerns about the secondary invasion of *M bovis* into the lesion cannot be refuted. This viewpoint is not met for either individual or herd-level studies.

Biologic Gradient (Dose–Response Relationship)

Greater exposure should generally lead to greater incidence of the effect. However, in some cases, the mere presence of the factor can trigger the effect. In other cases, an inverse proportion is observed: greater exposure leads to lower incidence.

The concept of a biologic gradient has not been explored for M bovis or M bovoculi, and this viewpoint is difficult to establish for pathogens. Generally, this viewpoint is used for toxins, that is, more smoking leads to more severe disease or rapid disease development. To assess this viewpoint, it would be necessary to document that exposure to more M bovis or M bovoculi is associated with either more severe lesions or more rapid development of lesions. This would require the ability to conduct a study that quantified M bovis or M bovoculi exposure. No such studies have been reported in the peer-reviewed literature. Another example of biologic gradient might occur if ecological studies were available to show that M bovis or M bovoculi prevalence was correlated with high IBK incidence at the herd level. Such an association would be evidence of a biologic gradient at the ecological level. Such studies are not publicly available. This viewpoint is not met for either individual or herd-level studies.

Plausibility

A plausible mechanism between cause and effect is helpful (but Hill noted that knowledge of the mechanism is limited by current knowledge). For M bovis, the viewpoint of plausibility is certainly meet with respect to toxins. These data are reviewed elsewhere in this issue. The toxins produced by M bovis suggested that the organism could plausibly cause IBK. Similarly, it seems plausible that M bovoculi could also cause IBK simply by its close relationship to M bovis. However, this viewpoint is only a springboard to research that should provide evidence for the other viewpoints. Researchers are exceptionally good at the concept of plausibility, and yet the relationship are not causal.

Coherence

Coherence between epidemiologic and laboratory findings increases the likelihood of an effect. However, Hill[3] noted that "… lack of such [laboratory] evidence cannot nullify the epidemiologic effect on associations." Coherence refers to the concept that observation studies and laboratory studies triangulate, that is, point in the same direction toward causation. For example, observational studies of smoking and lung cancer were coherent with studies of lung pathology in smokers compared with nonsmokers and consistent with laboratory studies suggesting that cigarette contents were toxic to respiratory cells.[3] Specifically, Hill[3] identified that the histopathologic of the bronchial epithelium of smokers and the isolation from cigarette smoke of factors carcinogenic for the skin of laboratory animals contributed to the concept of coherence for lung cancer and smoking.[3] Similarly, with the Zika virus, many studies documented the adverse effects of Zika virus on the growing neurosphere and brain organoid using human neural stem cells and Zika virus's ability to induce death of human neural cells.[4–7] It seems that this viewpoint was used by Hill[3] to refer to findings from in vitro studies and models of disease in the nontarget species.

For M bovis, the evidence for the coherence is perhaps some of the strongest for causal inference of M bovis in IBK. This evidence is well-reviewed in John Dustin Loy and colleagues' article, "Component causes of IBK - Non-Moraxella organisms in the epidemiology of Infectious Bovine keratoconjunctivitis," in this issue.[20] Loy and coworkers conclude, "The causal role of M bovis is clear, where the presence of virulence factors that facilitate colonization (pili) and host cytotoxicity (RTX toxins) are well characterized, and IBK pathology has been reproduced in many models." Numerous studies have documented the presence of toxins in *M bovis* that adhere and harm ocular cells.[21–24] For *M bovoculi*, the evidence is largely absent. Again this information is well-reviewed John Dustin Loy and colleagues' article, "Component causes of IBK - Non-Moraxella organisms in the epidemiology of Infectious Bovine keratoconjunctivitis," in this issue.[20] Compared with *M bovis*, there is scant evidence that *M bovoculi* can adhere to and harm ocular cells in in vitro studies.[25] Several studies have documented in noncattle animal models that eyes inoculated with *M bovis* are at risk of developing IBK-like lesions when the model includes corneal injury either by scarification or ultraviolet light.[26–28]

Experiment

Occasionally it is possible to appeal to experimental evidence. Based on Hill's[3] discussion, experimental evidence referred to "natural" experiments on the population.[3] Hill[3] refers to studies that suggest a deliberate intervention to add or remove the exposure resulting in a change in incidence.[3] However, several of the authors of the Zika virus reviews interpreted this viewpoint as referring to animal models.[7] In veterinary science, models of disease can be conducted in the species of interest, something that would not occur to Hill. Therefore, models of disease in the species of interest are discussed here in the experimentation viewpoint.

Veterinary scientists can conduct deliberate challenge experimental studies in the species of interest. This viewpoint provides the most robust evidence base for reaching a causal conclusion that *M bovis* causes IBK. Numerous challenge studies have documented that cattle inoculated with *M bovis* are at risk of developing IBK-like lesions, especially when the model includes corneal injury either by scarification or ultraviolet light.[28–37] Since these challenge studies were conducted the late 1960s, few studies have been conducted that evaluated causation. Instead, the models became the standard for preliminary investigations of IBK vaccines and treatment options. Since *M bovoculi* was reported as a putative causal organism only one challenge has been published (based on a PubMed search: "*Moraxella bovoculi*" AND cattle AND [experiment OR challenge OR model] AND "*Moraxella bovis*" AND cattle AND [experiment OR challenge OR model]). This sole publicly available study that assessed experimental induction of IBK with *M bovoculi* failed to document that *M bovoculi* could induce disease. In a three-arm scarification challenge study, calves were challenged with either *M bovis*, *M bovoculi*, or no organism challenge. The results were as follows: 9 of 10 *M bovis*–challenged calves (90%), 0 of 10 (0%) *M bovoculi*–challenged calves, and 1 of 11 (90%) control calves developed corneal ulcerations consistent with IBK in the scarified eyes. The absence of corneal ulcerations in *M bovoculi* BAA-1259-challenged calves suggests it is not a causal organism for IBK in this model. Furthermore, the pathogenicity of this ATCC strain has not been established. Consistent corneal ulceration development in the *M bovis*–challenged group demonstrates the ability of the model to induce IBK ulcers.

The only other data from experimental studies for the causal role of *M bovoculi* are minimal and not supportive. A 2007 report in the US Department of Agriculture CRIS database of an unpublished study reported similar results. The authors reported using a UV light model to induce IBK in two control calves and four challenge calves. No corneal ulcers were induced in the *M bovoculi* group or the control group as the authors reported: "Results of this study suggest that challenge with *Moraxella bovoculi* isolate 237 caused conjunctivitis in calves. The ultraviolet output of the sunlamps that were used to cause corneal irritation (a previously documented model of causing corneal ulceration in calves with *Moraxella bovis*) is suspected to be less than optimal, and therefore this study will need to be revised and repeated with new sunlamps. As of this writing, the ability of *Moraxella bovoculi* to cause corneal ulceration in calves still needs to be determined."[a] The results of this small prior trial support the concept that *M bovoculi* is not causal. However, the study omitted a positive control group that would document the ability of the model to induce disease, meaning that it was not possible to differentiate between the conclusion that the model was ineffective or the organism was not causal.

The other possible area of experimental is either natural or deliberate removal of exposure associated with reduced disease. This evidence could be in the form of removal or reduction of *M bovis* from the environment, which is not feasible, or protection of the individual from *M bovis* using vaccination. As reviewed Gabriele Maier and colleagues' article, "The evidence base for prevention of Infectious Bovine Keratoconjunctivitis through vaccination," in this issue, no field-based clinical trials of autogenous or commercial vaccines have documented the protection of animals from IBK after vaccination directed at *M bovis* or *M bovoculi*.[16,38–45] How this evidence can be used in causal inference is curious. If vaccination against *M bovis* (or *M bovoculi*) did prevent IBK, such a finding would provide some evidence toward a causal role. However, failure to document that a vaccine is protective does not refute a causal role of *M bovis* or *M bovoculi*. Failure to document a protective effect may occur because the vaccine does not target the correct organism in the particular herd or the vaccine is just not presenting the right antigen to a suitable immune component.

Analogy

Analogy usually refers to the situation where the proposed mechanism of disease is similar to another known cause, such as when reports of calves with hydranencephaly and cerebellar hypoplasia were associated with seropositivity to bovine viral diarrhea virus. That the bovine viral diarrhea virus was a *Pestivirus* of the family Flaviviridae and border disease in lambs (or hairy shaker disease lambs) have similar lesions and are also caused by a *Pestivirus* was considered to support a causal role of bovine viral diarrhea virus.[46] It is challenging to separate analogy from plausibility. This viewpoint is likely to be met for *M bovis* and *M bovoculi* both, because there is analogous evidence that *Moraxella* spp cause ocular lesions, although more commonly conjunctivitis, rather than corneal ulcer in children.[47–50]

SUMMARY

In veterinary science, it is considered well established that *M bovis* is a cause of IBK, so it might be surprising that many of the viewpoints that Bradford Hill provided do not explicitly support a causal role. However, this is usually a result of a lack of evidence rather than refuting evidence. For *M bovis*, the most robust support from a causal role in IBK comes from the experimental evidence and coherence of laboratory studies with that experimental evidence. Observationally, the evidence is weak. Most observational evidence comes from the isolation of *M bovis* from IBK lesions. These data points had been used as supportive of a causal role until the advent of *M bovoculi*. The data from *M bovoculi* have complicated causal inference for IBK. Although there is an abundance of evidence that *M bovoculi* can be recovered by lesions with IBK,

---

[a] USDA CRIS report-full history http://cris.nifa.usda.gov/cgi-bin/starfinder/6263/crisassist.txt Accession No: 0211472 Subfile: CRIS ProjNo: CA-V-VME-4013-AH-301 Agency: NIFA CALV Proj Type: AnimalHealth.

there has not been additional evidence that supports the role of *M bovoculi*, that is, there is almost no laboratory evidence that is coherent with the observational studies, and there are no publicly available experimental challenge studies that support a causal role for *M bovoculi* and IBK.

REFERENCES

1. Evans AS. Causation and disease: the Henle-Koch postulates revisited. Yale J Biol Med 1976;49(2):195.
2. Hosainzadegan H, Khalilov R, Gholizadeh P. The necessity to revise Koch's postulates and its application to infectious and non-infectious diseases: a mini-review 2020;39(2):218.
3. Hill AB. The environment and disease: association or causation? Proc R Soc Med 1965;58(5):295–300.
4. Kleber de Oliveira W, Cortez-Escalante J, De Oliveira WT, et al. Increase in reported prevalence of microcephaly in infants born to women living in areas with confirmed zika virus transmission during the first trimester of pregnancy—Brazil, 2015. MMWR Morb Mortal Wkly Rep 2016;65(9):242–7.
5. Awadh A, Chughtai AA, Dyda A, et al. Does zika virus cause microcephaly: applying the Bradford Hill viewpoints. PLoS Curr 2017;9. ecurrents.outbreaks.2fced6e886074f886076db886162a886000d4940133b.
6. Frank C, Faber M, Stark K. Causal or not: applying the Bradford Hill aspects of evidence to the association between Zika virus and microcephaly. EMBO Mol Med 2016;8(4):305–7.
7. Rasmussen SA, Jamieson DJ, Honein MA, et al. Zika virus and birth defects: reviewing the evidence for causality. N Engl J Med 2016;374(20):1981–7.
8. Shepard TH. "Proof" of human teratogenicity. Teratology 1994;50(2):97–8.
9. Kundi M. Causality and the interpretation of epidemiologic evidence. Environ Health Perspect 2006;114(7):969–74.
10. Cox LA Jr. Modernizing the Bradford Hill criteria for assessing causal relationships in observational data. Crit Rev Toxicol 2018;48(8):682–712.
11. Shimonovich M, Pearce A, Thomson H, et al. Assessing causality in epidemiology: revisiting Bradford Hill to incorporate developments in causal thinking. Eur J Epidemiol 2020. [Epub ahead of print].
12. O'Connor AM, Shen HG, Wang C, et al. Descriptive epidemiology of *Moraxella bovis*, *Moraxella bovoculi* and *Moraxella ovis* in beef calves with naturally occurring infectious bovine keratoconjunctivitis (Pinkeye). Vet Microbiol 2012;155(2):374–80.
13. Lepper AW, Barton IJ. Infectious bovine keratoconjunctivitis: seasonal variation in cultural, biochemical and immunoreactive properties of *Moraxella bovis* isolated from the eyes of cattle. Aust Vet J 1987;64(2):33–9.
14. Wilcox GE. The aetiology of infectious bovine keratoconjunctivitis in Queensland. 1. *Moraxella bovis*. Aust Vet J 1970;46(9):409–14.
15. Pearce N. Effect measures in prevalence studies. Environ Health Perspect 2004; 112(10):1047–50.
16. Cullen JN, Engelken TJ, Cooper V, et al. Randomized blinded controlled trial to assess the association between a commercial vaccine against *Moraxella bovis* and the cumulative incidence of infectious bovine keratoconjunctivitis in beef calves. J Am Vet Med Assoc 2017;251(3):345–51.
17. Hughes DE, Pugh GW Jr. A five-year study of infectious bovine keratoconjunctivitis in a beef herd. J Am Vet Med Assoc 1970;157(4):443–51.

18. Schnee C, Heller M, Schubert E, et al. Point prevalence of infection with *Mycoplasma bovoculi* and *Moraxella* spp. in cattle at different stages of infectious bovine keratoconjunctivitis. Vet J 2015;203(1):92–6.
19. McMullen C, Alexander TW, Orsel K, et al. Progression of nasopharyngeal and tracheal bacterial microbiotas of feedlot cattle during development of bovine respiratory disease. Vet Microbiol 2020;248:108826.
20. Loy JD, Hille M, Maier G, et al. Component causes of IBK: the role of *Moraxella* spp. in the epidemiology of infectious bovine keratoconjunctivitis. In: Veterinary Clinics of North America, Food animal Practices. 2021.
21. Rogers DG, Cheville NF, Pugh GW Jr. Pathogenesis of corneal lesions caused by *Moraxella bovis* in gnotobiotic calves. Vet Pathol 1987;24(4):287–95.
22. Kagonyera GM, George LW, Munn R. Cytopathic effects of *Moraxella bovis* on cultured bovine neutrophils and corneal epithelial cells. Am J Vet Res 1989; 50(1):10–7.
23. Kagonyera GM, George LW, Munn R. Light and electron microscopic changes in corneas of healthy and immunomodulated calves infected with *Moraxella bovis*. Am J Vet Res 1988;49(3):386–95.
24. Angelos JA, Hess JF, George LW. An RTX operon in hemolytic *Moraxella bovis* is absent from nonhemolytic strains. Vet Microbiol 2003;92(4):363–77.
25. Cerny HE, Rogers DG, Gray JT, et al. Effects of *Moraxella (Branhamella) ovis* culture filtrates on bovine erythrocytes, peripheral mononuclear cells, and corneal epithelial cells. J Clin Microbiol 2006;44(3):772–6.
26. Lepper AW, Power BE. Infectivity and virulence of Australian strains of *Moraxella bovis* for the murine and bovine eye in relation to pilus serogroup sub-unit size and degree of piliation. Aust Vet J 1988;65(10):305–9.
27. Nakazawa M, Sakuta Y, Nemoto H. Relationship between biological properties of *Moraxella bovis* and its virulence for mice. Natl Inst Anim Health Q (Tokyo) 1979; 19(4):132–3.
28. Pugh GW Jr, Hughes DE, Schulz VD. The pathophysiological effects of *Moraxella bovis* toxins on cattle, mice and guinea pigs. Can J Comp Med 1973;37(1):70–8.
29. Vogelweid CM, Miller RB, Berg JN, et al. Scanning electron microscopy of bovine corneas irradiated with sun lamps and challenge exposed with *Moraxella bovis*. Am J Vet Res 1986;47(2):378–84.
30. Chandler RL, Turfrey BA, Smith K. Laboratory model for infectious bovine keratoconjunctivitis: the pathogenicity of different strains of *Moraxella bovis*, pathology and ultrastructural observations. Res Vet Sci 1983;35(3):277–84.
31. Chandler RL, Turfrey BA, Smith K. Development of a laboratory animal model for infectious bovine keratoconjunctivitis. Res Vet Sci 1982;32(1):128–30.
32. Kopecky KE, Pugh GW Jr, Hughes DE. Wavelength of ultraviolet radiation that enhances onset of clinical infectious bovine keratoconjunctivitis. Am J Vet Res 1980; 41(9):1412–5.
33. Pugh GW Jr, Hughes DE. Comparison of the virulence of various strains of *Moraxella bovis*. Can J Comp Med 1970;34(4):333–40.
34. Pugh GW Jr, Hughes DE, Packer RA. Bovine infectious keratoconjunctivitis: interactions of *Moraxella bovis* and infectious bovine rhinotracheitis virus. Am J Vet Res 1970;31(4):653–62.
35. Hughes DE, Pugh GW Jr, McDonald TJ. Ultraviolet radiation and *Moraxella bovis* in the etiology of bovine infectious keratoconjunctivitis. Am J Vet Res 1965; 26(115):1331–8.
36. Hughes DE, Pugh GW Jr, McDonald TJ. Experimental bovine infectious keratoconjunctivitis caused by sunlamp irradiation and *Moraxella bovis* infection:

resistance to re-exposure with homologous and heterologous *Moraxella bovis*. Am J Vet Res 1968;29(4):829–33.

37. Pugh GW Jr, Hughes DE. Experimental bovine infectious keratoconjunctivitis caused by sunlamp irradiation and *Moraxella bovis* infection: correlation of hamolytic ability and pathogenicity. Am J Vet Res 1968;29(4):835–9.

38. Smith PC, Blankenship T, Hoover TR, et al. Effectiveness of two commercial infectious bovine keratoconjunctivitis vaccines. Am J Vet Res 1990;51(7):1147–50.

39. Angelos JA, Hess JF, George LW. Prevention of naturally occurring infectious bovine keratoconjunctivitis with a recombinant *Moraxella bovis* cytotoxin-ISCOM matrix adjuvanted vaccine. Vaccine 2004;23(4):537.

40. George LW, Borrowman AJ, Angelos JA. Effectiveness of a cytolysin-enriched vaccine for protection of cattle against infectious bovine keratoconjunctivitis. Am J Vet Res 2005;66(1):136–42.

41. Angelos JA, Gohary KG, Ball LM, et al. Randomized controlled field trial to assess efficacy of a *Moraxella bovis* pilin-cytotoxin-*Moraxella bovoculi* cytotoxin subunit vaccine to prevent naturally occurring infectious bovine keratoconjunctivitis. Am J Vet Res 2012;73(10):1670–5.

42. O'Connor A, Cooper V, Censi L, et al. A 2-year randomized blinded controlled trial of a conditionally licensed *Moraxella bovoculi* vaccine to aid in prevention of infectious bovine keratoconjunctivitis in Angus beef calves. J Vet Intern Med 2019; 33(6):2786.

43. O'Connor AM, Brace S, Gould S, et al. A randomized clinical trial evaluating a farm-of-origin autogenous *Moraxella bovis* vaccine to control infectious bovine keratoconjunctivis (pinkeye) in beef cattle. J Vet Intern Med 2011;25(6):1447–53.

44. Funk L, O'Connor AM, Maroney M, et al. A randomized and blinded field trial to assess the efficacy of an autogenous vaccine to prevent naturally occurring infectious bovine keratoconjunctivis (IBK) in beef calves. Vaccine 2009;27(34): 4585–90.

45. Angelos JA, Lane VM, Ball LM, et al. Recombinant *Moraxella bovoculi* cytotoxin-ISCOM matrix adjuvanted vaccine to prevent naturally occurring infectious bovine keratoconjunctivitis. Vet Res Commun 2010;34(3):229–39.

46. Radostits OM, Littlejohns IR. New concepts in the pathogenesis, diagnosis and control of diseases caused by the bovine viral diarrhea virus. Can Vet J 1988; 29(6):513–28.

47. Epling J. Bacterial conjunctivitis. BMJ Clin Evid 2012;2012.

48. LaCroce SJ, Wilson MN, Romanowski JE, et al. *Moraxella* nonliquefaciens and *M. osloensis* are important moraxella species that cause ocular infections. Microorganisms 2019;7(6).

49. Leung AKC, Hon KL, Wong AHC, et al. Bacterial conjunctivitis in childhood: etiology, clinical manifestations, diagnosis, and management. Recent Pat Inflamm Allergy Drug Discov 2018;12(2):120–7.

50. Verduin CM, Hol C, Fleer A, et al. *Moraxella* catarrhalis: from emerging to established pathogen. Clin Microbiol Rev 2002;15(1):125–44.

Component Causes of Infectious Bovine Keratoconjunctivitis - The Role of *Moraxella* Species in the Epidemiology of Infectious Bovine Keratoconjunctivitis

John Dustin Loy, DVM, PhD, DACVM[a],*, Matthew Hille, DVM[a],
Gabriele Maier, DVM, MPVM, PhD, DACVPM[b], Michael L. Clawson, PhD[c]

KEYWORDS

- Infectious bovine keratoconjunctivitis • *Moraxella bovis* • *Moraxella bovoculi*
- *Moraxella ovis* • MALDI-TOF MS • Genomics • Pathogenesis

KEY POINTS

- *Moraxella bovis* can cause infectious bovine keratoconjunctivitis (IBK).
- The role of *M bovoculi* in IBK is not fully understood.
- *M bovis* and *M bovoculi* appear to undergo genetic recombination with each other or other members of the *Moraxellaceae*.
- Recombination complicates their classification and potential role(s) in IBK pathogenesis.
- MALDI-TOF MS is used to identify *M bovis*, 2 major strains or genotypes of *M bovoculi*, *M ovis*, and other members of the *Moraxellaceae*.
- Classification and determination of pathogenesis potential within *Moraxella* species may be better understood through whole genome sequencing.

INTRODUCTION

Bacterial pathogens have been associated with infectious bovine keratoconjunctivitis (IBK) or pinkeye, from some of the earliest descriptions of the disease. While investigating outbreaks of keratitis contagiosia in Nebraska cattle, one of the first

[a] Nebraska Veterinary Diagnostic Center, School of Veterinary Medicine and Biomedical Sciences, University of Nebraska-Lincoln, 4040 East Campus Loop North 115Q NVDC, Lincoln, NE 68583-0907, USA; [b] Department of Population Health & Reproduction, School of Veterinary Medicine, University of California Davis, 1 Shields Avenue, VM3B, Davis, CA 95616, USA; [c] US Meat Animal Research Center, USDA Agriculture Research Service, Clay Center, 844 Road 313, Clay Center, NE 68933, USA
* Corresponding author.
E-mail address: jdloy@unl.edu

Vet Clin Food Anim 37 (2021) 279–293
https://doi.org/10.1016/j.cvfa.2021.03.004
0749-0720/21/© 2021 Elsevier Inc. All rights reserved.

documented reports of IBK, Billings described dense clusters of coccoid bacteria in corneal lesions. The organisms were subsequently isolated in pure culture; however, he was unsuccessful in reproducing the disease in healthy animals.[1] These early observations and experiments highlight some of the discoveries, knowledge gaps, and controversy that remain after 120 years of research on the causality of IBK. This article will focus on bacterial causes of IBK, specifically members of the genus *Moraxella*, likely the same organisms Billings observed in 1898.

Moraxella bovis (M bovis) is the most common bacterial species associated with the disease and appears well suited to cause IBK. *M bovis* possesses numerous adherence and colonization factors, secretes toxins and enzymes that damage bovine cells, and utilizes various mechanisms to avoid immune recognition and enable persistence in hosts. *M bovis* is the only pathogen to have reproduced IBK-like ocular lesions in various experimental models, including in gnotobiotic calves, indicating that it is capable of inducing disease in the absence of other potential pathogens and with cell-free supernatants, which is evidence for the role of secreted exotoxins in the pathogenicity of IBK.[2–4] For other members of the genus, primarily *Moraxella bovoculi (M bovoculi)*, direct causality appears less clear, as reproduction of the disease following experimental infection with pure culture has not yet been achieved.[5] However, the presence of virulence factors in *M bovoculi* similar in structure and function to *M bovis*, along with recent genomic data showing recombination between the 2 species, highlights the complexity of IBK pathogenesis and possible interactions. The role these pathogens play in causing and/or contributing to IBK is reviewed, including virulence factors, studies on causality, recent findings using genomics and mass spectrometry, and detection and differentiation of these organisms in clinical samples.

The Genus Moraxella

The genus *Moraxella* represents the type genus within the larger family *Moraxellaceae*.[6] *Moraxella* are gram-negative rods or cocci, which are oxidase and usually catalase positive.[7] There are 22 validly published species, most of which are parasites or commensals of mucous membranes of mammals.[7,8] *Moraxella* is among the most abundant organisms in the upper respiratory and ocular microbiome, and overall abundance of this genus was not found to be associated with risk of IBK in 1 study.[9,10] Three species within the genus have been studied in relation to IBK, and include *M bovis*, *M bovoculi*, and *Moraxella* (formerly *Branhamella* and *Neisseria*) *ovis (M ovis)*. There is likely taxonomic overlap between *M ovis* and *M bovoculi*. In the authors' view, *M ovis* is rare and mostly absent from ocular cultures of cattle, and reports or descriptions of *M ovis* from the eyes of cattle prior to the recognition of *M bovoculi* are likely *M bovoculi*. Both species can appear identical if utilizing only biochemical testing.[11] This view agrees with several large prevalence or descriptive epidemiology studies that found low numbers or no *M ovis* in cattle ocular cultures that have occurred since the description of *M bovoculi* as a separate species using polymerase chain reaction (PCR) or other nonbiochemical methods for identification.[12–15]

MORAXELLA BOVIS- VIRULENCE FACTORS
Repeats in Toxin

Exotoxins are a hallmark of many bacterial pathogens and repeats-in-toxin (RTX) type toxins found in numerous pathogenic bacteria. RTX toxins are thought to have originated in members of the *Pasteurellaceae*, and subsequently disseminated among other bacteria through horizontal gene transfer.[16] RTX toxins are large, pore-forming proteins with a common structure of glycine and aspartate-rich repeats, and are secreted via a type I secretion system, a transporter necessary to enable secretion of toxin from the cytoplasm to the environment.[17] RTX toxins include *Escherichia coli* alpha hemolysin, *Mannheimia haemolytica* leukotoxin, and the Apx family of *Actinobacillus pleuropneumoniae* toxins.[18,19] *M bovis* RTX toxin, also called hemolysin, cytolysin, or cytotoxin, reacts with monoclonal antibodies to other RTX toxins and forms pores in bovine erythrocytes, demonstrating similarity in structure and function to other RTX toxins.[20,21] *M bovis* RTX toxin is toxic to bovine neutrophils and corneal epithelium, but not human neutrophils.[22,23] The host cell receptor for *M bovis* cytotoxin has not been definitively determined, but other closely related toxins bind to B_2 integrins on leukocytes, and some, like *M haemolytica* leukotoxin, bind to a host-specific CD18 signal peptide region.[18,24,25] This property makes the toxin highly specific to certain cell types, which likely leads to clinical signs observed in associated diseases. For example, *M bovis* RTX toxin is a necessary and sufficient virulence factor for IBK, where toxin-rich supernatants from hemolytic strains have been shown to reproduce IBK-like lesions in vivo, and nonhemolytic strains and supernatants are avirulent or nontoxic.[26,27] The RTX toxin is expressed in some *M bovis* strains in part by a gene (*mbx*A), which is absent in nonhemolytic strains and under the control of an operon, which forms a pathogenicity island.[28–30] Activity of the toxin is neutralized by rabbit antiserum raised against the carboxy terminus of *mbx*A.[28] In addition to *mbx*A, the RTX operon genes include *mbx*C (toxin activation protein), *mbx*B (transport protein), and *mbx*D (transport protein) and a flanking protein related to TolC, a secretion protein similar to other RTX toxin operons (type 1 secretion system).[17,29] A high degree of conservation in *mbx*A has been observed among isolates from diverse geographic origins, which makes this a potential vaccine antigen target.[31,32]

MORAXELLA BOVIS PILI

Type IV pili, also known as fimbriae or attachment pili, are small structural protein fibers made up of pilin proteins that serve numerous functions.[33] In *M bovis,* they facilitate attachment to corneal epithelium, a process that is inhibited by pili-specific antiserum. Pili are a necessary virulence factor, and strains lacking pili are unable to adhere and therefore cannot cause disease.[34–36] Inhibition of adherence by pili-specific antiserum is serogroup specific, with at least 7 different serogroups described.[37] Protection from IBK using pili-based vaccines was shown to be serotype specific in 1 study.[38] Selection and maintenance of pili in culture through selection and passage of agar-corroding colonies with pili enabled successful challenge and colonization models, as pili expression appears to decrease upon passage (**Fig. 1**).[39–41] The isolation frequency of piliated colony types from cattle changes based on seasonality and has been observed to positively correlate with levels of UV radiation.[42] *M bovis* also expresses 2 mutually exclusive forms of pilin, called Q (quick) and I (intermediate), in addition to serotype level variation conferred by pili.[43,44] The expression of pili is reversible and under the control of an inversion region under a single promoter.[44,45] The Q pili form has been shown to be more effective at binding to corneal epithelium than both I pili forms and non-piliated strains.[46] *M bovis* selectively attaches, presumably through pili, to dark cells in the cornea, those that are older and devoid of membrane ridges called microplicae, when viewed by scanning electron microscopy; the number of these cells is increased by UV light.[47] This observation has led to the hypothesis that other environmental factors or coinfections that increase the proportion of dark cells in the cornea may potentially enhance the ability of *M bovis* to colonize.[4,48,49] Pili are also involved in the formation of biofilms on both biotic and abiotic surfaces; this formation of biofilms seems to confer greater resistance to lysozyme.[50,51]

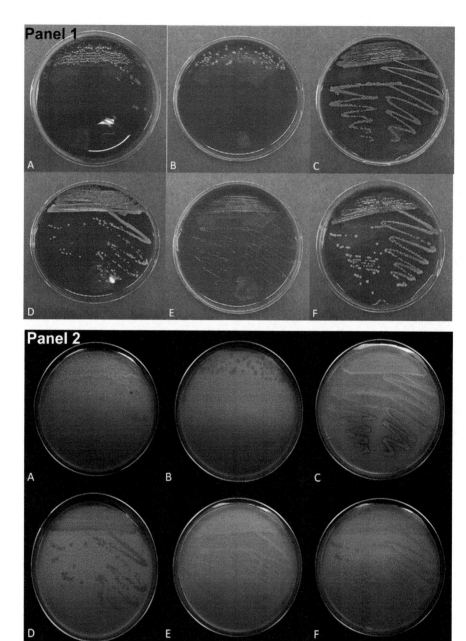

Fig. 1. Panel 1. Differences in *Moraxella* colony phenotypes. Images were captured after 48-hour growth in 5% CO_2 atmosphere on trypticase soy agar with 5% defibrinated bovine erythrocytes. (*A*) Strain Epp 63, *M bovis*, RTX +, beta hemolysis. (*B*) Isolate 0131, *M bovis* recombinant, RTX +, beta hemolysis. (*C*) Isolate Mb58081, *M bovoculi*, genotype 1, RTX +, beta hemolysis. (*D*) Isolate Mb58090, *M bovoculi*, genotype 1, RTX –, gamma hemolysis. (*E*) Mb58000, *M bovoculi*, genotype 1, RTX +, stop codon at codon 70 of PilA gene (no pili production), beta hemolysis. (*F*) Mb 68,535, *M bovoculi*, genotype 2, RTX -, gamma hemolysis. Panel 2. Same plates as panel 1 with backlighting to visualize hemolysis. (Images by Matthew Hille and Justin Lowery.)

MORAXELLA BOVIS OTHER POTENTIAL VIRULENCE FACTORS

M bovis possesses an outer membrane (OM) that consists of at least 3 distinct types of lipooligosaccharide (LOS), which are uniquely devoid of heptose.[52,53] The biologic role of LOS for *M bovis* was demonstrated, as mutants with truncated LOS (shortened and less functional) had increased susceptibility to the bactericidal activity of bovine serum, decreased adherence to mammalian cells, and increased sensitivity to detergents and some antibiotics.[54] Some *M bovis* strains also express a capsular polysaccharide.[54,55] OM proteins are the first line of defense against host immune defenses, and these studies provide supportive evidence that in *M bovis* they may serve as virulence factors.

M bovis strains produce an array of hydrolytic enzymes, which facilitate the breakdown of host protein, lipids, nucleic acids, carbohydrate and fat molecules into their simplest units, and therefore can cause damage to ocular tissues. These include esterases, lipases, phosphoamidase, phosphatase, and hyaluronidase. *M bovis* strains can also hydrolyze casein, produce fibrinolysin, and are agarolytic.[56] Some strains express and secrete phospholipase, which is conserved and has been considered by some as a potential vaccine antigen.[57] Other strains carry a plasmid encoding filamentous haemagglutinin-like proteins (*flp*A and *flp*B), which may facilitate host colonization, similar to virulence factors found in *Bordetella pertussis*.[58] Iron acquisition is a critical function for pathogens to replicate and maintain infections, as iron is tightly regulated in the host environment. Some *M bovis* strains also possess iron-repressible outer membrane proteins similar to the human pathogen *N meningitidis* (*lrp*A)[59] and have robust iron acquisition machinery, including fur homologues, and are capable of acquiring iron from bovine lactoferrin (lbp) and transferrin (tbp).[60,61]

STUDIES ON *MORAXELLA BOVIS* AND CAUSALITY

Experimental studies have definitively demonstrated that *M bovis* can cause IBK-like lesions compared with uninfected controls.[5,62–64] However, insults to the cornea such as ultraviolet (UV) radiation or corneal scarification may be necessary in experimental infection studies to induce IBK.[5,65] Lesions have also been produced in the absence of corneal insults, and whether they are required may depend on the infectious dose or the strain virulence and immune status of the host.[63] Experimental infections with some strains appear to be enhanced by coinoculation with *M bovoculi*.[66] Evidence for the causal role of *M bovis* in IBK came through experimental infections with strains of known virulence in gnotobiotic calf models, which have reproduced clinical and lesions consistent with IBK, including histopathological changes in the cornea and conjunctiva in the absence of other factors such as trauma or coinfections with other bacterial species.[3,4,67] Purified fractions of *M bovis* cell-free supernatants were shown to reproduce IBK lesions in calves, implying a role for a specific excreted *M bovis* virulence factor to cause IBK, which we now understand to be the RTX toxin encoded by *mbx*A.[2]

In field studies, *M bovis* is often isolated from IBK-affected cattle, but it is also found in normal healthy eyes, with variations in isolation rates observed depending on seasonality and animal age.[42,68,69] One study showed high prevalence of isolation of *M bovis* in the absence of other agents in outbreaks that were diverse in space and time, but did not include cultures from nondiseased eyes for comparison.[70] A study of an outbreak during winter, winter pinkeye, had a high prevalence of *M bovis* isolated in the absence of other agents, and the isolates were able to reproduce IBK in calves, but this study also did not culture healthy eyes for comparison.[71] More recent studies using PCR methods showed only a weak temporal association between *M bovis* detection and IBK in naturally occurring outbreaks of IBK.[14] The observation that *M bovis* is isolated from nonclinical animals at similar rates as those from IBK cases has been documented numerous times in epidemiologic studies, thus complicating the picture of a single infectious agent that is alone necessary and sufficient for causality.[72,73]

The mechanism for why discrepancies between the presence of *M bovis* and clinical cases of IBK are observed could be comparable to what is understood about bovine respiratory disease (BRD). Many of the pathogens associated with BRD can be isolated from the respiratory tract of healthy animals. Immunomodulatory effects of common bovine viral infections or stress allow for these opportunistic pathogens to replicate, invade deeper into the respiratory tract, secrete toxins, and cause disease.[74] Likewise, *M bovis* may only be able to cause IBK if other conditions are met, such as stress, physical damage, UV radiation, or face fly irritation. Also, with BRD there are well-defined strains, or genotypes, of *M haemolytica* that differ by their armament of virulence factors and outer membrane proteins, and by their association with BRD.[75,76] The same could be true for *M bovis* and IBK, because of changes in alleles throughout the genome that alter or enhance virulence. More detailed discussion about causal models for IBK is available elsewhere in this issue.

MORAXELLA BOVIS GENOMICS

Genetic diversity among *M bovis* has been examined through DNA fingerprinting with enterobacterial repetitive intergenic consensus (ERIC), and random amplified polymorphic DNA (RAPD).[53,77] Recently, the first complete whole-genome sequence of the Epp63 strain, used in many studies, was published.[78] Aside from having known virulence factors including an RTX operon, multiple pilin and prepilin genes, and other genes involved with adhesion, the Epp63 genome has numerous repetitive regions. These include 2 repeat regions associated with CRISPR and 5800 repeat regions consisting of dinucleotide to decanucleotide units, ranging in size from 8 to 422 bases. The repeats are located throughout the genome, either in noncoding regions, coding regions, or both, which suggests that *M bovis* may employ slipped strand mispairing coupled to phase variation as a way to adapt to particular niche environments including changing host immune responses directed at select *M bovis* antigens. Multiple pathogens employ this technique, which may enable *M bovis* strains to vary their pathogenicity by the phase state of their genomes.[79] On a practical level, multiple repeat regions probably explain why there is a paucity of fully assembled *M bovis* genomes in public databases at present, as short reads of a sequence commonly produced by most sequencing technologies would not span these large repeat regions, which would interfere with the assembly of a complete *M bovis* genome. Additional complete genomes will be required to understand *M bovis* genomic diversity better, as well as strain pathogenicity or lack thereof, and the extent of recombination between *M bovis* and other members of the *Moraxellaceae*.

MORAXELLA BOVOCULI
Virulence Factors

Several virulence factors homologous to those found in *M bovis* have been found within *M bovoculi*, which provides partial support for the hypothesis that it may play a role in IBK pathogenesis, despite not having been able to replicate IBK-like lesions in experimental infections. The 2 most significant homologous virulence factors are a complete RTX operon and type IV pilin proteins.[80,81] The *mbvA* gene, responsible for the RTX toxin (also called cytotoxin A) within *M bovoculi* is highly conserved with

99.3% nucleotide and 98.8% corresponding amino acid homology within the species.[32] Similar to *M bovis*, the RTX toxin of *M bovoculi* is necessary for hemolytic activity (**Fig. 2**).[80,82] Although the RTX toxins produced by *M bovis* and *M bovoculi* are similar in structure and function, within an *in vitro* model using bovine erythrocytes, polyclonal serum raised against *M bovoculi* RTX toxin did not neutralize corresponding *M bovis* toxin activity encoded by *mbxA*, but did neutralize *M ovis* RTX toxin, thus indicating sufficient differences between *M bovis* and *M bovoculi* toxins in structure to require additional immune responses.[80] Some of these RTX-related operon sequences found in *M bovoculi* demonstrate what appears to be interspecies mosaicism, where recombination with *M bovis* RTX-related sequences (*mbvB* and *mbvD*) is apparent in some sequences.[83]

Sequence analysis of *M bovoculi* pilin (*pilA*) appears to be substantially different than that of *M bovis*, with as little as 38% sequence homology between the 2 species.[81] However, *M bovoculi* pilin sequences show limited intraspecies diversity in contrast to *M bovis*.[83,84] The large diversity between species suggests that any cross-protection to pilin epitopes would be minimal. The potential importance of the few variable regions within *M bovoculi* pilin sequences is unknown. If these variable regions prove to be important clinically, it could explain the failures thus far to produce disease experimentally and/or provide an effective immune response using a limited number of isolates, as the variable regions may be important determinants of initial ocular colonization and disease initiation, as observed with *M bovis*.

Like *M bovis*, *M bovoculi* has also been shown to form biofilms on abiotic surfaces such as polystyrene microplates.[51] Biofilms have a well-established association with disease severity in numerous microbial diseases of people and animals.[85,86] Biofilm formation is variable within *M bovoculi*, and also could potentially contribute to variation in virulence. For example, the type strain of *M bovoculi* (BAA1259) has moderate biofilm-forming capacity, where more recently isolated field strains of *M bovoculi* used in the study had stronger biofilm-forming capability.[51] Given the relatedness of the species, the reliance on type IV pilus for biofilm formation would seem likely, but this has not been examined within *M bovoculi*.

CHALLENGE MODELS

In 1 study, *M bovoculi* did not cause IBK in conventionally reared calves, even though a hemolytic isolate representing the type strain was used for the challenge. In this same study, controls using *M bovis* strain Epp63 did cause disease consistent with

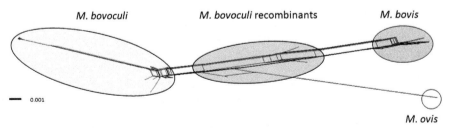

Fig. 2. Neighbor-joining network made in SplitsTree of full length 16S sequences. The network contains 18 *M bovis* sequences (contained in the blue ellipse and described by Robbins and colleagues), 253 *M bovoculi* non-recombinant and recombinant sequences (contained in the yellow and green ellipses, respectively, and described by Dickey and colleagues, GenBank# SRP070887) and 2 *M ovis* sequences (contained in the white circle, GenBank # AF005186 and NR_028670). The scale bar equals substitutions per site.

IBK using the same randomized and blinded challenge model.[5] These findings are in agreement with a smaller study from 25 years prior in which *M ovis* (likely *M bovoculi*) did not cause corneal lesions in a small group of calves.[87] Gould and colleagues[60] recognized this older study was inadequate because of a lack of a positive control, meaning it was not possible to determine if the organism did not cause disease or the model was incapable of causing disease. Regardless, *M bovoculi* has not demonstrated a causal relationship to IBK under experimental conditions. However, genomic diversity within *M bovoculi* further complicates interpreting this challenge work, as only limited strains have been used for experimental inoculations.[83,88]

MORAXELLA BOVOCULI AND CAUSALITY

Despite not having shown to reproduce the disease experimentally, a hallmark of infectious disease causation in veterinary science, there are some findings that support a potential contributive or associative role for *M bovoculi* in IBK pathogenesis. Prior to the characterization of *M bovoculi*, isolates classified as *M ovis* (likely *M bovoculi*) were isolated three times more often than *M bovis* from clinical samples of IBK cases submitted to a diagnostic laboratory.[82] More recently, *M bovoculi* was the only bacteria isolated from most (64%) of individual animal cases of IBK over a 4-year timeframe with only 22% of cases isolating only *M bovis*.[13] In this same study, the authors found when examining cases where more than 1 bacterial species was isolated, *M bovoculi* and *M bovis* were isolated from 74% and 32% of cases, respectively.[13] Another study utilizing real-time PCR detection on diagnostic laboratory submissions found similar results, where 75.9% of samples (136/179) had *M bovoculi* detected.[89] In studies looking at prevalence of *Moraxella,* one study showed that only the detection of *M bovoculi* by PCR methods was associated with clinical signs of IBK. This same study also showed that prevalence of *M bovoculi* may be associated with likelihood of undergoing an acute IBK outbreak.[68] Another study showed the recovery of *M bovoculi* and *M bovis* was more frequent from eyes with IBK lesions than unaffected eyes.[14] It also showed that calves infected with *M bovis* had a higher subsequent risk of developing IBK than calves infected with *M bovoculi*.[14] Caution should be taken to avoid overinterpretation of postlesion microbiological data, which does not establish temporality between presence of pathogens and occurrence of lesions.[5] Documenting that exposure occurs before disease is essential for establishing causation in future studies.

MORAXELLA BOVOCULI GENOMICS

M bovoculi has recently been classified into 2 major strain types, or genotypes (1 and 2), based on whole-genome sequencing of over 200 isolates.[83,88] The genotypes differ in several ways. Both genotype 1 and 2 *M bovoculi* have been isolated from the eyes of cattle without IBK, while only genotype 1 *M bovoculi*, which includes the type strain, has been isolated and identified from the eyes of cattle with IBK. However, the frequency and potential role, or lack thereof, of genotype 2 *M bovoculi* in IBK remain poorly understood. Genotype 2 *M bovoculi* has only recently been described, and isolates may have been inadvertently misclassified as non-*bovoculi Moraxella* in the past based on a PCR typing method instead of biochemical for *M bovoculi* that was developed prior to their discovery.[88,90] The PCR-based typing method only identifies genotype 1 strains, as genotype 2 strains do not contain the restriction enzyme binding site targeted in the method to distinguish *M bovoculi* from *M ovis* and other *Moraxella* species.[83,90,91] Thus, the difference between the genotypes in IBK-positive or -negative eyes needs to be tested in more studies that do not have biases in isolate identification. Recently, a MALDI-TOF biomarker method, which uses mass spectrometry peaks that are genotype specific to classify *M bovoculi* isolates, was developed that would make these data easier to generate, as these instruments are now available in many diagnostic laboratories.[92]

Genotype 1 *M bovoculi* appears to be more diverse than genotype 2. Over 127,000 SNPs have been identified within and across the 2 *M bovoculi* genotypes, with over 80% characterizing diversity exclusively in genotype 1 strains.[83] The 2 genotypes also appear to differ in their RTX profiles. To date, no genotype 2 strains have been found to have an RTX operon versus 85% of genotype 1 strains isolated from IBK eyes that do, including the type strain.[83] Thus, current studies suggest that *M bovoculi* genotypes may differ in their propensity to cause or contribute to the development of IBK, with genotype 1 isolates more likely to have RTX, and extensive genetic diversity, and genotype 2 isolates having genomic profiles more consistent with commensals.

CLASSIFICATION OF *MORAXELLA BOVIS* AND *MORAXELLA BOVOCULI*

MALDI-TOF assays that enable identification of *M bovis* and the 2 genotypes of *M bovoculi* may be improved or enhanced as more is learned about the 2 species and the extent of recombination that may have taken place between them. There is compelling evidence that *M bovoculi* has recombinant 16S rDNA alleles (see **Fig. 2**) that were possibly acquired from *M bovis*, and *M bovis* has recombinant alleles within the internal transcribed spacer region of the ribosomal locus.[91] Given the high conservation of the ribosomal locus throughout the evolution of bacteria, it is not unexpected that these species have extensive recombination elsewhere throughout their genomes.[83] This observation challenges assignment of IBK causality, as these mixed chimeric genomes may not be easily assigned to 1 species. However, it is possible to distinguish *M bovis*, *M bovoculi*, and *M bovoculi* recombinants from each other with full-length 16S rDNA sequences (see **Fig. 2**). Full-genome sequences will ultimately be much more powerful in classifying these bacteria as an identity -by -state combination of alleles acquired through vertical descent and horizontal lateral gene transfer events. The same may be true for other members of the *Moraxellaceae*, and methods that classify members of this family using full, or particularly partial 16S sequences, may be shown to conflate members of the family. Examples include *M ovis* and members of the closely related genus *Psychrobacter,* which are also found in cattle and have been isolated from bovine eye swabs by the authors.[93,94]

SUMMARY AND FUTURE WORK

Whole-genome sequencing of *M bovis* and *M bovoculi* strains isolated from the eyes of cattle with or without IBK, followed by genome comparisons, may reveal core genetic determinants that are necessary for virulence and further understanding of the diversity and contributions of these organisms to IBK.

CLINICS CARE POINTS- DIAGNOSIS AND ESTABLISHMENT OF *MORAXELLA* ETIOLOGY IN INFECTIOUS BOVINE KERATOCONJUNCTIVITIS

- Determining the etiology in individual outbreaks is challenging, because *Moraxella* species have been isolated from cases of IBK and normal eyes, and the isolation of an agent after the appearance of a lesion does not establish causation.
- For microbiological sample collection, the ocular conjunctival sac is aggressively swabbed to culture for pathogens while avoiding contamination. Use of flocked

swabs in liquid transport media offers enhanced collection and release of bacteria into the media.[95]
- False-negative culture results can occur if there is contamination or multiple pathogens.
- PCR as a culture independent modality can be useful, although caveats and challenges related to classification and misclassification of *Moraxella*, as discussed, also apply to PCR diagnostic methods.
- A multiplexed real-time PCR is available that targets the toxin genes for *M bovis* (*mbx*A) and *M bovoculi* (*mbv*A).[89] Similar approaches for bovine respiratory disease pathogens have been shown to increase co-detections over culture alone.[96]
- The authors routinely see case submissions from field outbreaks of IBK where only *M bovoculi* is isolated by culture, but similar levels (Ct values) of *M bovis* toxin genes are detected by real-time PCR, which indicates the potential for false-negative *M bovis* cultures.
- Newly developed MALDI-TOF assays provide quick, accurate, and economic methods to identify *Moraxella* species from culture. These methods also allow differentiation of *M bovoculi* isolates traditionally associated with disease versus those that likely represent normal flora.[91,92]

DISCLOSURE

The authors have nothing to disclose.

REFERENCES

1. Billings FS. Keratitis contagiosa in cattle. Nebr Agric Exp Station Bull 1889;10: 246–52.
2. Beard MK, Moore LJ. Reproduction of bovine keratoconjunctivitis with a purified haemolytic and cytotoxic fraction of Moraxella bovis. Vet Microbiol 1994;42(1): 15–33.
3. Rogers DG, Cheville NF, Pugh GW Jr. Pathogenesis of corneal lesions caused by Moraxella bovis in gnotobiotic calves. Vet Pathol 1987;24(4):287–95.
4. Chandler R, Turfrey B, Smith K, et al. Virulence of Moraxella bovis in gnotobiotic calves. Vet Rec 1980;106(16):364–5.
5. Gould S, Dewell R, Tofflemire K, et al. Randomized blinded challenge study to assess association between Moraxella bovoculi and infectious bovine keratoconjunctivitis in dairy calves. Vet Microbiol 2013;164(1–2):108–15.
6. Rossau R, Van landschoot A, Gillis M, et al. Taxonomy of Moraxellaceae fam. nov., a new bacterial family to accommodate the genera Moraxella, Acinetobacter, and Psychrobacter and related organisms. Int J Syst Evol Microbiol 1991;41(2):310–9.
7. Moraxella. Bergey's manual of systematics of archaea and bacteria. 2012. p. 1-17.
8. Parte AC, Sardà Carbasse J, Meier-Kolthoff JP, et al. List of prokaryotic names with standing in nomenclature (LPSN) moves to the DSMZ. Int J Syst Evol Microbiol 2020;70:5607–12.
9. Cullen JN, Lithio A, Seetharam AS, et al. Microbial community sequencing analysis of the calf eye microbiota and relationship to infectious bovine keratoconjunctivitis. Vet Microbiol 2017;207:267–79.
10. Nicola I, Cerutti F, Grego E, et al. Characterization of the upper and lower respiratory tract microbiota in Piedmontese calves. Microbiome 2017;5(1):152.

11. Angelos JA. *Moraxella bovoculi* and infectious bovine keratoconjunctivitis: cause or coincidence? Vet Clin North Am Food Anim Pract 2010;26(1):73–8, table of contents.

12. Maboni G, Gressler LT, Espindola JP, et al. Differences in the antimicrobial susceptibility profiles of *Moraxella bovis, M bovoculi* and *M ovis*. Braz J Microbiol 2015;46(2):545–9.

13. Loy JD, Brodersen BW. *Moraxella* spp. isolated from field outbreaks of infectious bovine keratoconjunctivitis: a retrospective study of case submissions from 2010 to 2013. J Vet Diagn Invest 2014;26(6):761–8.

14. O'Connor AM, Shen HG, Wang C, et al. Descriptive epidemiology of *Moraxella bovis, Moraxella bovoculi* and *Moraxella ovis* in beef calves with naturally occurring infectious bovine keratoconjunctivitis (pinkeye). Vet Microbiol 2012;155(2–4): 374–80.

15. Angelos JA, Spinks PQ, Ball LM, et al. *Moraxella bovoculi* sp. nov., isolated from calves with infectious bovine keratoconjunctivitis. Int J Syst Evol Microbiol 2007; 57(Pt 4):789–95.

16. Frey J, Kuhnert P. RTX toxins in *Pasteurellaceae*. Int J Med Microbiol 2002;292(3): 149–58.

17. Linhartova I, Osicka R, Bumba L, et al. RTX toxins: a review. In: Gopalakrishnakone P, Stiles B, Alape-Girón A, et al, editors. Microbial toxins. Dordrecht: Springer Netherlands; 2016. p. 1–29.

18. Frey J. RTX toxins of animal pathogens and their role as antigens in vaccines and diagnostics. Toxins (Basel) 2019;11(12):719.

19. Welch RA. Pore-forming cytolysins of gram-negative bacteria. Mol Microbiol 1991;5(3):521–8.

20. Gray JT, Fedorka-Cray PJ, Rogers DG. Partial characterization of a *Moraxella bovis* cytolysin. Vet Microbiol 1995;43(2–3):183–96.

21. Clinkenbeard KD, Thiessen AE. Mechanism of action of *Moraxella bovis* hemolysin. Infect Immun 1991;59(3):1148–52.

22. Kagonyera GM, George LW, Munn R. Cytopathic effects of *Moraxella bovis* on cultured bovine neutrophils and corneal epithelial cells. Am J Vet Res 1989; 50(1):10–7.

23. Kagonyera GM, George L, Miller M. Effects of *Moraxella bovis* and culture filtrates on 51Cr-labeled bovine neutrophils. Am J Vet Res 1989;50(1):18–21.

24. Shanthalingam S, Srikumaran S. Intact signal peptide of CD18, the beta-subunit of beta2-integrins, renders ruminants susceptible to Mannheimia haemolytica leukotoxin. Proc Natl Acad Sci U S A 2009;106(36):15448–53.

25. Li J, Clinkenbeard KD, Ritchey JW. Bovine CD18 identified as a species specific receptor for *Pasteurella haemolytica* leukotoxin. Vet Microbiol 1999;67(2):91–7.

26. Beard MK, Moore LJ. Reproduction of bovine keratoconjunctivitis with a purified haemolytic and cytotoxic fraction of *Moraxella bovis*. Vet Microbiol 1994;42(1): 15–33.

27. Pugh GW Jr, Hughes DE. Experimental bovine infectious keratoconjunctivitis caused by sunlamp irradiation and *Moraxella bovis* infection: correlation of haemolytic ability and pathogenicity. Am J Vet Res 1968;29(4):835–9.

28. Angelos JA, Hess JF, George LW. Cloning and characterization of a *Moraxella bovis* cytotoxin gene. Am J Vet Res 2001;62(8):1222–8.

29. Angelos JA, Hess JF, George LW. An RTX operon in hemolytic *Moraxella bovis* is absent from nonhemolytic strains. Vet Microbiol 2003;92(4):363–77.

30. Hess JF, Angelos JA. The *Moraxella bovis* RTX toxin locus mbx defines a pathogenicity island. J Med Microbiol 2006;55(4):443–9.

31. Angelos JA, Ball LM. Relatedness of cytotoxins from geographically diverse isolates of *Moraxella bovis*. Vet Microbiol 2007;124(3–4):382–6.

32. Farias LDA, Maboni G, Matter LB, et al. Phylogenetic analysis and genetic diversity of 3′ region of rtxA gene from geographically diverse strains of *Moraxella bovis*, *Moraxella bovoculi* and *Moraxella ovis*. Vet Microbiol 2015;178(3):283–7.

33. Giltner CL, Nguyen Y, Burrows LL. Type IV pilin proteins: versatile molecular modules. Microbiol Mol Biol Rev 2012;76(4):740–72.

34. Moore LJ, Rutter JM. Attachment of *Moraxella bovis* to calf corneal cells and inhibition by antiserum. Aust Vet J 1989;66(2):39–42.

35. Jayappa HG, Lehr C. Pathogenicity and immunogenicity of piliated and nonpiliated phases of *Moraxella bovis* in calves. Am J Vet Res 1986;47(10):2217–21.

36. Gil-Turnes C. Hemagglutination, autoagglutination and pathogenicity of *Moraxella bovis* strains. Can J Comp Med 1983;47(4):503–4.

37. Moore LJ, Lepper AW. A unified serotyping scheme for *Moraxella bovis*. Vet Microbiol 1991;29(1):75–83.

38. Lepper AWD, Moore LJ, Atwell JL, et al. The protective efficacy of pili from different strains of *Moraxella bovis* within the same serogroup against infectious bovine keratoconjunctivitis. Vet Microbiol 1992;32(2):177–87.

39. Lepper AW. Pink Eye of Cattle. In: Butcher B, editor. Of vets, viruses and vaccines: the story of CSIRO's Animal Health Research Laboratory. Collingwood, Vic: CSIRO; 2000. p. 194–9.

40. Ruehl WW, Marrs CF, Fernandez R, et al. Purification, characterization, and pathogenicity of *Moraxella bovis* pili. The J Exp Med 1988;168(3):983–1002.

41. Pedersen KB, Frøholm LO, Bøvre K. Fimbriation and colony type of *Moraxella bovis* in relation to conjunctival colonization and development of keratoconjunctivitis in cattle. Acta Pathol Microbiol Scand B Microbiol Immunol 1973;80B(6):911–8.

42. Lepper AW, Barton IJ. Infectious bovine keratoconjunctivitis: seasonal variation in cultural, biochemical and immunoreactive properties of *Moraxella bovis* isolated from the eyes of cattle. Aust Vet J 1987;64(2):33–9.

43. Marrs CF, Schoolnik G, Koomey JM, et al. Cloning and sequencing of a *Moraxella bovis* pilin gene. J Bacteriol 1985;163(1):132–9.

44. Marrs CF, Ruehl WW, Schoolnik GK, et al. Pilin-gene phase variation of *Moraxella bovis* is caused by an inversion of the pilin genes. J Bacteriol 1988;170(7): 3032–9.

45. Fulks KA, Marrs CF, Stevens SP, et al. Sequence analysis of the inversion region containing the pilin genes of *Moraxella bovis*. J Bacteriol 1990;172(1):310–6.

46. Ruehl WW, Marrs C, Beard MK, et al. Q pili enhance the attachment of *Moraxella bovis* to bovine corneas in vitro. Mol Microbiol 1993;7(2):285–8.

47. Vogelweid CM, Miller RB, Berg JN, et al. Scanning electron microscopy of bovine corneas irradiated with sunlamps and challenge exposed with *Moraxella bovis*. Am J Vet Res 1986;47(2):378–84.

48. Jackman SH, Rosenbusch RF. In vitro adherence of *Moraxella bovis* to intact corneal epithelium. Curr Eye Res 1984;3(9):1107–12.

49. Chandler RL, Bird RG, Smith MD, et al. Scanning electron microscope studies on preparations of bovine cornea exposed to *Moraxella bovis*. J Comp Pathol 1983; 93(1):1–8.

50. Prieto C, Serra DO, Martina P, et al. Evaluation of biofilm-forming capacity of *Moraxella bovis*, the primary causative agent of infectious bovine keratoconjunctivitis. Vet Microbiol 2013;166(3):504–15.

51. Ely VL, Vargas AC, Costa MM, et al. *Moraxella bovis, Moraxella ovis* and *Moraxella bovoculi*: biofilm formation and lysozyme activity. J Appl Microbiol 2019; 126(2):369–76.

52. De Castro C, Grice ID, Daal TM, et al. Elucidation of the structure of the oligosaccharide from wild type *Moraxella bovis* Epp63 lipooligosaccharide. Carbohydr Res 2014;388:81–6.

53. Prieto CI, Aguilar OM, Yantorno OM. Analyses of lipopolysaccharides, outer membrane proteins and DNA fingerprints reveal intraspecies diversity in *Moraxella bovis* isolated in Argentina. Vet Microbiol 1999;70(3–4):213–23.

54. Singh S, Grice ID, Peak IR, et al. The role of lipooligosaccharide in the biological activity of *Moraxella bovis* strains Epp63, Mb25 and L183/2, and isolation of capsular polysaccharide from L183/2. Carbohydr Res 2018;467:1–7.

55. Wilson JC, Hitchen PG, Frank M, et al. Identification of a capsular polysaccharide from *Moraxella bovis*. Carbohydr Res 2005;340(4):765–9.

56. Frank SK, Gerber JD. Hydrolytic enzymes of *Moraxella bovis*. J Clin Microbiol 1981;13(2):269–71.

57. Farn JL, Strugnell RA, Hoyne PA, et al. Molecular characterization of a secreted enzyme with Phospholipase B Activity from *Moraxella bovis*. J Bacteriol 2001; 183(22):6717–20.

58. Kakuda T, Sarataphan N, Tanaka T, et al. Filamentous-haemagglutinin-like protein genes encoded on a plasmid of *Moraxella bovis*. Vet Microbiol 2006;118(1): 141–7.

59. Kakuda T, Oishi D, Tsubaki S, et al. Molecular cloning and characterization of a 79-kDa iron-repressible outer-membrane protein of *Moraxella bovis*. FEMS Microbiol Lett 2003;225(2):279–84.

60. Kakuda T, Oishi D, Tsubaki S, et al. Cloning and characterization of the fur gene from *Moraxella bovis*. Microbiol Immunol 2003;47(6):411–7.

61. Yu R-H, Schryvers AB. Bacterial lactoferrin receptors: insights from characterizing the Moraxella bovis receptors. Biochem Cell Biol 2002;80(1):81–90.

62. Aikman JG, Allan EM, Selman IE. Experimental production of infectious bovine keratoconjunctivitis. Vet Rec 1985;117(10):234–9.

63. Chandler RL, Baptista PJ, Turfrey B. Studies on the pathogenicity of *Moraxella bovis* in relation to infectious bovine keratoconjunctivitis. J Comp Pathol 1979; 89(3):441–8.

64. Henson JB, Grumbles LC. Infectious bovine keratoconjunctivitis. I. Etiology. Am J Vet Res 1960;21:761–6.

65. Weech GM, Renshaw HW. Infectious bovine keratoconjunctivitis: bacteriologic, immunologic, and clinical responses of cattle to experimental exposure with *Moraxella bovis*. Comp Immunol Microbiol Infect Dis 1983;6(1):81–94.

66. Rosenbusch RF. Influence of mycoplasma preinfection on the expression of *Moraxella bovis* pathogenicity. Am J Vet Res 1983;44(9):1621–4.

67. Rogers DG, Cheville NF, Pugh GW Jr. Conjunctival lesions caused by *Moraxella bovis* in gnotobiotic calves. Vet Pathol 1987;24(6):554–9.

68. Schnee C, Heller M, Schubert E, et al. Point prevalence of infection with *Mycoplasma bovoculi* and *Moraxella* spp. in cattle at different stages of infectious bovine keratoconjunctivitis. Vet J 2015;203(1):92–6.

69. Bartenslager AC, Althuge ND, Loy JD, et al. Longitudinal assessment of the bovine ocular bacterial community dynamics in calves. Anim Microbiome 2021; 3(1):16.

70. Wilcox GE. The aetiology of infectious bovine keratoconjunctivitis in Queensland 1. *Moraxella bovis*. Aust Vet J 1970;46(9):409–14.

71. Pugh GW Jr, Hughes DE. Bovine infectious keratoconjunctivitis: *Moraxella bovis* as the sole etiologic agent in a winter epizootic. J Am Vet Med Assoc 1972; 161(5):481–6.
72. Barber DM, Jones GE, Wood A. Microbial flora of the eyes of cattle. Vet Rec 1986; 118(8):204–6.
73. Pugh GW Jr, McDonald TJ. Identification of bovine carriers of *Moraxella bovis* by comparative cultural examinations of ocular and nasal secretions. Am J Vet Res 1986;47(11):2343–5.
74. Mosier D. Review of BRD pathogenesis: the old and the new. Anim Health Res Rev 2014;15(2):166–8.
75. Clawson ML, Murray RW, Sweeney MT, et al. Genomic signatures of *Mannheimia haemolytica* that associate with the lungs of cattle with respiratory disease, an integrative conjugative element, and antibiotic resistance genes. BMC Genomics 2016;17(1):982.
76. Clawson ML, Schuller G, Dickey AM, et al. Differences between predicted outer membrane proteins of genotype 1 and 2 *Mannheimia haemolytica*. BMC Microbiol 2020;20(1):250.
77. Comin HB, Domingues R, Gaspar EB, et al. Genetic differences among *Moraxella bovis* and *Moraxella bovoculi* isolates from infectious bovine keratoconjunctivitis (IBK) outbreaks in southern Brazil. Genet Mol Biol 2020;43(2): e20180380-e20180380.
78. Loy JD, Dickey AM, Clawson ML. Complete genome sequence of *Moraxella bovis* strain Epp-63 (300), an etiologic agent of infectious bovine keratoconjunctivitis. Microbiol Resour Announc 2018;7(8):e01004–18.
79. van der Woude MW, Baumler AJ. Phase and antigenic variation in bacteria. Clin Microbiol Rev 2004;17(3):581–611, table of contents.
80. Angelos JA, Ball LM, Hess JF. Identification and characterization of complete RTX operons in *Moraxella bovoculi* and *Moraxella ovis*. Vet Microbiol 2007; 125(1–2):73–9.
81. Calcutt MJ, Foecking MF, Martin NT, et al. Draft genome sequence of *Moraxella bovoculi* strain 237T (ATCC BAA-1259T) isolated from a calf with infectious bovine keratoconjunctivitis. Genome Announc 2014;2(3):e00612–4.
82. Cerny HE, Rogers DG, Gray JT, et al. Effects of *Moraxella (Branhamella) ovis* culture filtrates on bovine erythrocytes, peripheral mononuclear cells, and corneal epithelial cells. J Clin Microbiol 2006;44(3):772–6.
83. Dickey AM, Schuller G, Loy JD, et al. Whole genome sequencing of *Moraxella bovoculi* reveals high genetic diversity and evidence for interspecies recombination at multiple loci. PLoS One 2018;13(12):e0209113.
84. Angelos JA, Clothier KA, Agulto RL, et al. Relatedness of type IV pilin PilA amongst geographically diverse *Moraxella bovoculi* isolated from cattle with infectious bovine keratoconjunctivitis. J Med Microbiol 2021;70:001293.
85. Costerton JW, Stewart PS, Greenberg EP. Bacterial biofilms: a common cause of persistent infections. Science 1999;284(5418):1318–22.
86. Abdullahi UF, Igwenagu E, Mu'azu A, et al. Intrigues of biofilm: a perspective in veterinary medicine. Vet World 2016;9(1):12–8.
87. Rosenbusch RF, Ostle AG. *Mycoplasma bovoculi* infection increases ocular colonization by *Moraxella ovis* in calves. Am J Vet Res 1986;47(6):1214–6.
88. Dickey AM, Loy JD, Bono JL, et al. Large genomic differences between *Moraxella bovoculi* isolates acquired from the eyes of cattle with infectious bovine keratoconjunctivitis versus the deep nasopharynx of asymptomatic cattle. Vet Res 2016;47(1):31.

89. Zheng W, Porter E, Noll L, et al. A multiplex real-time PCR assay for the detection and differentiation of five bovine pinkeye pathogens. J Microbiol Methods 2019; 160:87–92.
90. Angelos JA, Ball LM. Differentiation of *Moraxella bovoculi* sp. nov. from other coccoid *Moraxellae* by the use of polymerase chain reaction and restriction endonuclease analysis of amplified DNA. J Vet Diagn Invest 2007;19(5):532–4.
91. Robbins KJ, Dickey AM, Clawson ML, et al. Application and evaluation of the matrix-assisted laser desorption ionization time of flight (MALDI-TOF) mass spectrometry method to identify *Moraxella bovoculi* and *Moraxella bovis* isolates from cattle. J Vet Diagn Invest 2018;30(5):739–42.
92. Hille M, Dickey A, Robbins K, et al. Rapid differentiation of *Moraxella bovoculi* genotypes 1 and 2 using MALDI-TOF mass spectrometry profiles. J Microbiol Methods 2020;173:105942.
93. Holman DB, Timsit E, Amat S, et al. The nasopharyngeal microbiota of beef cattle before and after transport to a feedlot. BMC Microbiol 2017;17(1):70.
94. Shen HG, Gould S, Kinyon J, et al. Development and evaluation of a multiplex real-time PCR assay for the detection and differentiation of *Moraxella bovis, Moraxella bovoculi* and *Moraxella ovis* in pure culture isolates and lacrimal swabs collected from conventionally raised cattle. J Appl Microbiol 2011;111(5): 1037–43.
95. Van Horn KG, Audette CD, Tucker KA, et al. Comparison of 3 swab transport systems for direct release and recovery of aerobic and anaerobic bacteria. Diagn Microbiol Infect Dis 2008;62(4):471–3.
96. Loy JD, Leger L, Workman AM, et al. Development of a multiplex real-time PCR assay using two thermocycling platforms for detection of major bacterial pathogens associated with bovine respiratory disease complex from clinical samples. J Vet Diagn Invest 2018;30(6):837–47.

Component Causes of Infectious Bovine Keratoconjunctivitis—Non-Moraxella Organisms in the Epidemiology of Infectious Bovine Keratoconjunctivitis

John Dustin Loy, DVM, PhD[a],*, Kristin A. Clothier, DVM, PhD[b],
Gabriele Maier, DVM, MPVM, PhD, DACVPM[c]

KEYWORDS

- IBK • Pink eye • Infectious bovine keratoconjunctivitis, *Mycoplasma bovoculi*
- *Ureaplasma* • Bovine herpesvirus • Listeria • Chlamydia

KEY POINTS

- Non-Moraxella organisms are associated with infectious bovine keratoconjunctivitis (IBK).
- *Mycoplasma bovoculi* can cause conjunctivitis and has a potential role in IBK pathogenesis.
- Other Non-Mycoplasma agents can cause disease that resembles IBK but is clinically different.
- Genomics and molecular technology are advancing research in this area.
- Classification and determination of pathogenesis potential of these organisms may be better understood through metagenomics and whole genome sequencing.

INTRODUCTION

Historically the role of bacterial organisms associated with infectious bovine kerato-conjunctivitis (IBK) has fallen to members of the genus *Moraxella* (see John Dustin Loy and colleagues' article, "Component causes of IBK - The Role of *Moraxella* spp. in the epidemiology of Infectious Bovine Keratoconjunctivitis," in this issue.).

[a] Nebraska Veterinary Diagnostic Center, School of Veterinary Medicine and Biomedical Sciences, University of Nebraska-Lincoln, Lincoln, NE, USA; [b] Department of Pathology, Microbiology, and Immunology, California Animal Health and Food Safety Laboratory System, School of Veterinary Medicine, University of California Davis, 620 W. Health Sciences Drive, Davis, CA 95616, USA; [c] Department of Population Health & Reproduction, School of Veterinary Medicine, University of California Davis, 1 Shields Avenue, VM3B, Davis, CA 95616, USA
* Corresponding author. 4040 East Campus Loop N. 115Q NVDC, Lincoln, NE 68583-0907.
E-mail address: jdloy@unl.edu

Vet Clin Food Anim 37 (2021) 295–308
https://doi.org/10.1016/j.cvfa.2021.03.005
0749-0720/21/© 2021 Elsevier Inc. All rights reserved.

However, there are numerous other pathogens that have been described in association with either outbreaks or clinical cases of IBK with and without an association with *Moraxella*. The most significant of these include members of the genus *Mycoplasma*, specifically *Mycoplasma bovis* and *Mycoplasma bovoculi*, which have long been found associated with ocular infections in cattle. Other less understood potential pathogens include intracellular organisms such as *Chlamydia* spp. Viral causes such as bovine herpesvirus have also been associated with IBK. Other ocular diseases, including those caused by *Listeria monocytogenes*, may often have some clinical overlap with IBK-like diseases. Although none of these agents has strong support as a direct cause of IBK, there is evidence that infections with some may predispose animals to IBK. The role of these agents in association with IBK or IBK-like disease is reviewed later, including virulence factors, studies on causality, immune responses, and importantly detection and interpretation of diagnostic findings of these organisms in IBK cases.

Mycoplasma

Members of the genus *Mycoplasma* are small pleomorphic bacteria that lack a cell wall, are nutritionally fastidious, have a limited metabolism, and are composed of 124 species.[1] Most of the well-studied members of the genus are human or animal pathogens; however, about half of these exist as commensals or opportunistic pathogens that colonize fish, reptiles, and birds in addition to mammals.[1] There are at least 13 members of the genus *Mycoplasma* that infect cattle, and these include those that cause respiratory, reproductive, mastitis, systemic diseases, and ocular infections.[2] *Mycoplasma* is one of the most abundant genera present in the bovine upper respiratory tract.[3–5] Evaluations of microbiota from calves with and without disease indicated that animals with otitis and pneumonia have a greater abundance of *Mycoplasma* sp than those without; and all conditions had a greater *Mycoplasma* sp abundance than healthy cohorts.[6] *Mycoplasma* has been studied by using 16S ribosomal sequencing to look at microbial communities within the bovine eye. Among, the top 10 genera identified, *Mycoplasma* showed a higher mean relative abundance in the non-IBK controls (26.86%) compared with the IBK cases (18.29%).[7] An in vitro co-culture study conducted with human sinus epithelial cells and donor respiratory microbiota determined that the inclusion of TH-1 macrophages shifted the microbial abundance from *Corynebacterium* spp, *Staphylococcus* spp, and *Dolosigranulum* spp to an abundance of *Moraxella* spp and *Mycoplasma* spp, providing some insight into how mammalian host immune status may alter microbial composition.[8] Another recently published study evaluated the ocular microbiome in calves over time and showed that *Mycoplasma* spp were detected at all time points with variation in abundance over the preweaning period. Significant differences were also observed in microbial communities before and after clinical IBK disease, with both *Mycoplasmataceae* and *Moraxellaceae* families increasing post-IBK infection[9]; this indicates that *Mycoplasmas* are likely part of the ocular flora and may change over time and in response to IBK. The nutritionally fastidious nature of *Mycoplasmas* makes isolation and study in the laboratory challenging. Recovered isolates require additional characterization to identify the species isolated, which often is only performed in reference laboratories. However, with the advent of molecular techniques such as polymerase chain reaction (PCR) and gene sequencing, more tools are now available to aid researchers and veterinarians in the study and diagnosis of these infections, and future research using these techniques may establish more definitive roles for these agents in association with IBK. The lack of available tools such as vaccines and effective treatments has also impeded successful mitigation of the disease-causing *Mycoplasma* spp in animals, including cattle, and these areas deserve additional research attention.[10]

Mycoplasma bovoculi

M bovoculi was first described following an outbreak of IBK that yielded an isolate that was biochemically different from previously described *Mycoplasmas*.[11,12] *M bovoculi* has a specific requirement for sterol in the culture media; use of standard *Mycoplasma* media may not support recovery of this agent and cause false-negative results.[11]

Subsequent studies on microbial flora of cattle eyes have shown *M bovoculi* to be highly prevalent in normal calves, and asymptomatic infections can occur at an early age, with spread to other animals occurring over time, including over the winter months when vectors are at lower levels.[13] The average prevalence of *M bovoculi* in repeated samplings in this study was more than 45%, which, given the challenges in isolating this organism, may indicate a much higher true prevalence. Given the apparent high prevalence in cattle eyes, it is difficult to evaluate *M bovoculi's* contribution as a risk factor to IBK. It seems likely that *M bovoculi*, if a pathogen, is an opportunistic one that may contribute to disease instead of directly causing IBK. Some studies summarized later show mild or absent disease when *M bovoculi* is found alone but describe potentiation of disease when administered or found with other pathogens, such as *Moraxella bovis*. There may be synergism between *Mycoplasma* and *Moraxella* species; however, the exact mechanisms of such a process have not yet been described.

VIRULENCE FACTORS

Virulence factors and other characteristics of *M bovoculi* remain poorly understood. *M bovoculi* adheres to bovine epithelium in the absence of any specialized attachment structure and does not possess a capsule.[14] The adherence is tight and primarily to bovine conjunctival epithelial cells; organisms can be observed in infected animals when stained with specific florescent antibody.[15] Whole genome sequencing has been performed on the type strain of *M bovoculi*, which is the descendant of the original isolates used in the bacterial species description and which contains a 760,240 bp genome, 626 genes, and has 7 gene pairs potentially associated with adherence factors.[16] A novel contingency locus, that is, a region of hypermutable DNA, was also identified, which has an array of 5 genes that indicate phase variation and combinatorial expression patterns, which may be involved in host immune evasion or other host adaptations of *M bovoculi* outer membrane proteins.[17]

CLINICAL DISEASE

Clinically, cattle with *M bovoculi*–associated signs do not appear ill, but 10% to 90% may have a unilateral or bilateral ocular discharge and conjunctival hyperemia (**Fig. 1**).[18] Field investigations of "epizootic conjunctivitis," a disease entity considered clinically different from classic IBK, isolated primarily *M bovoculi* in 11 out of 19 Iowa farms from affected animals.[15] In a different study ocular samples from 6 herds with cattle showing signs of conjunctivitis yielded recovery of *M bovoculi* from 50% to 100% of cattle but no recovery from two herds without signs of conjunctivitis.[18] Experimental infection studies with *M bovoculi* inoculation report mild conjunctivitis, and some have shown infections with *M bovoculi* may predispose animals to Moraxella-induced IBK. For example, under experimental inoculation, calves exposed to *M bovoculi* (n = 6) and *Ureaplasma* spp (n = 6) developed conjunctivitis and lacrimation 3 to 4 days following challenge and were recovered 1 to 2 months after infection.[18] *M*

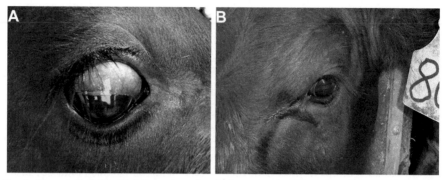

Fig. 1. (*A* and *B*) Calf with bilateral ocular discharge and mild conjunctivitis. PCR detected the presence of *Mycoplasma* spp in the absence of other agents. (*Courtesy of* Dr John Angelos, UC Davis.)

bovoculi was able to be reisolated from the bovine eye following co-challenge with *M bovis*.[19] Another study describes a potential enhancement effect of *M bovoculi* on *M bovis* challenge in colostrum-deprived calves, where those that received *M bovoculi* before *M bovis* challenge, 4/5 eyes developed conjunctivitis within 3 days versus only 1/3 that did not receive *M bovoculi* inoculation developing conjunctivitis.[20] However, the study lacked robust controls to evaluate the validity of this observed enhancement. Calves infected with *M bovoculi* in one study had longer colonization times and developed keratitis at higher rates when challenged with *M bovis* (n = 6/6 calves) when compared with those without mycoplasma exposure (0/4 calves).[21] *M bovoculi* also seemed to increase colonization levels of *Moraxella ovis* in calves. One study showed 0/3 calves had *M ovis* isolated from eyes 15 days after inoculation when compared with those that had been inoculated with *M bovoculi* before *M ovis* (3/3 calves). There were also significant differences in colony forming units/swab of *M ovis* isolated between these 2 treatment groups at earlier time points.[22] Even though several studies point toward a possible role of *Mycoplasma* in IBK, extrapolation of results from small experimental studies, which often lack blinding and randomization of study animals, requires confirmation of findings in field trials. Difficulty arises from the fact that prevalence of *M bovoculi* infection in eyes of cattle populations seems to be very high, which may actually obscure its potential role as a risk factor.

IMMUNITY

Immune responses to *M bovoculi* seem robust in recovered animals and include immunoglobulin A (IgA) in lacrimal and nasal secretions in addition to serum IgG and IgM and cellular immune responses.[23,24] Previous natural exposure to these organisms seems to provide protection against colonization. One study showed that in calves with evidence of prior *M bovoculi* colonization that were vaccinated and subsequently challenged, most cleared the organism by day 3 and all were negative by day 10 postchallenge. None of these animals showed evidence of conjunctivitis. In contrast, protection from *M bovoculi* challenge in gnotobiotic calves was not induced by administration of killed *M bovoculi* antigens (either from membrane extracts or killed whole organism); all animals developed conjunctivitis and had *M bovoculi* recovered throughout the study period (15 days).[24] *M bovoculi* strains have similar, but not identical, protein profiles, with antigenic differences apparent when evaluated by immunoblotting with serum from recovered calves. However, a 94 kDa outer membrane protein that seems antigenically identical across multiple strains and monoclonal antibodies raised against this protein interact with other *Mycoplasma* species.[25,26] Ocular challenge with *M bovoculi* seems to result in enhanced systemic natural killer (NK) cell activity as well as to induce NK migration into bovine eyes following acute infection.[27] A small study with 65 cattle from India found serum IgG antibodies that reacted to sonicated *M bovoculi* antigens in 44% of cattle with IBK and 15% of nonclinical cattle, indicating an association between immune response and clinical disease.[28]

EPIDEMIOLOGIC STUDIES

Some associations between the presence of *M bovoculi* and IBK have been found, but the evidence has to be interpreted with caution. Schnee and colleagues (2014) examined the point prevalence of IBK-associated pathogens in cattle from 4 different herds in Europe representing 4 different clinical stages of IBK. The investigators found that herds early in the course of IBK had a higher prevalence of *M bovoculi* detected by PCR than those recovering from or without clinical IBK and hypothesized that herds with higher *M bovoculi* prevalence are predisposed to acute outbreaks of IBK, possibly due to synergism with *Moraxella* spp. However, further studies are needed to confirm the findings of the cross-sectional study that may have been confounded by different breeds, housing types, or other management factors.[29] Other surveys indicate that the prevalence of *M bovoculi* in cattle eyes seems quite high in both clinical and nonclinical animals. One study mentioned earlier demonstrated that in a group of calves followed from 1 week to 15 months of age without clinical ocular disease, *M bovoculi* recovery rate by culture was initially low but increased over time with an overall prevalence of 45% in normal eyes.[13] Using a recently developed real-time PCR approach to detect IBK-associated pathogens, Zheng and colleagues found very high prevalence of *M bovoculi* in case submissions to a diagnostic laboratory (159/179; 88%). Although diagnostic submissions represent a biased sample, these results indicate that *M bovoculi* may be an underdetected component of IBK, and PCR testing may reveal it is present at high levels in diagnostic submissions and during outbreaks.[30]

Mycoplasma bovis

M bovis causes a wide array of significant bovine diseases that include pneumonia, mastitis, arthritis, otitis, and keratoconjunctivitis.[31] It possesses a variety of virulence factors involved in adherence, antigenic variation, host cell invasion, immune modulation, and biofilm formation.[31] *M bovis* has been shown to suppress host immunity via altered cytokine (interferon gamma and tumor necrosis factor alpha) expression, depressed oxidative burst from neutrophils, and suppressed lymphocyte proliferation.[31] In a retrospective study from a diagnostic reference laboratory in the United Kingdom, *M bovis* was the most frequently isolated *Mycoplasma* sp from bovine cases annually, representing 52% of all *Mycoplasmas* isolated from cattle over a 10-year period, which were primarily cultured from the lung or upper respiratory tract but also from eyes with IBK lesions.[32] *M bovis* was investigated as a cause in an outbreak of IBK in a beef herd that subsequently developed pneumonia and arthritis.[33] *M bovis* isolates were recovered during the outbreak investigation. All were identified as a single strain that had similarity to other European *M bovis* strains and possessed variable membrane surface lipoprotein (*vsp*) genes found in *M bovis* but not in other *Mycoplasma* spp.[34] *M bovis* has been reported in outbreaks of IBK in 1-year-old beef calves and a group of Holstein cattle in the absence of other pathogens.[35,36] *M bovis* has also been found in mixed *Mycoplasma* outbreaks of IBK (along with *M bovoculi*) in Holstein calves following morbidity with respiratory disease that had 30/40 affected.[37]

OTHER MYCOPLASMAS

Other *Mycoplasmas*, including *Mycoplasma bovirhinis* and *Mycoplasma bovigenitalium* in a mixed infection with bovine herpesvirus-1 (BoHV-1), have been reported associated with IBK. The significance of these findings is unknown because the role of the individual agents was not evaluated and the findings stem from a series of case reports.[38] Experimental inoculation of calves with *Mycoplasma conjunctivae* or *Acholeplasma laidlawii* did not result in IBK.[39]

Ureaplasma

Ureaplasma, originally classified as T-strain *Mycoplasmas*, are small pleomorphic bacteria that lack a cell wall and are very similar to *Mycoplasma*, with the exception of a requirement for urea for growth.[33] Similar to *Mycoplasma,* all of the members of the genus are obligate commensals or opportunistic pathogens of vertebrate hosts, primarily of mucosal surfaces. There are 7 species of *Ureaplasma*, and the species associated with bovine hosts is *U diversum*, of which there are 3 distinct serologic clusters.[40] Infections with *Ureaplasma* spp in cattle are typically associated with reproductive infections or fetal/neonatal pneumonia.[41] However, there have been some reports of *Ureaplasma*-associated ocular infections. Large colony and T-strain mycoplasmas (Ureaplasmas) have been isolated from ocular secretions, along with *M bovis* in cases of calves with IBK, but not in healthy calves; however, these results are from a single publication 50 years ago and have not been reproduced.[42] Case reports suggest fetal infections with *Ureaplasma spp* can induce extensive nonsuppurative conjunctivitis and goblet cell metaplasia throughout the eyelid epithelium.[43] *M bovoculi* and *Ureaplasma* sp have been recovered from outbreaks of epizootic conjunctivitis.[44] Inoculation of calves with *Ureaplasma* spp caused diffuse conjunctivitis and lacrimation, and organisms were able to be recovered from inoculated eyes up to 2 months postinfection.[18] Overall, the evidence for the role of *Ureaplasma* spp in IBK is limited at present to a few older studies, and its contribution to the disease complex is likely minor.

HERPESVIRUSES

Infections with BoHV-1, the causative agent of infectious bovine rhinotracheitis (IBR) can cause ocular disease that resembles IBK. Outbreaks of IBK-like diseases, some with an absence of corneal ulcers, had virus isolated from nasal and ocular secretions.[45–50] The virus isolated from early outbreaks was determined to be a herpesvirus indistinguishable from that causing IBR. In experimental infections, BoHV-1 produced conjunctivitis but not keratitis in challenged calves, thus indicating infection with this herpesvirus caused a disease distinct from IBK.[51,52] However, BoHV-1 has shown some association with IBK. Challenge with BoHV-1 alone in more recent studies caused conjunctivitis and blepharitis but not keratitis.[53] Pugh described higher prevalence of IBK in animals that were exposed to BoHV-1 before challenge with *M bovis* versus those that were exposed to BoHV-1 after *M bovis* challenge.[53] George and colleagues demonstrated that vaccination with a modified live IBR vaccine either intranasally or intraocularly increased lesion scores and isolation rates of *M bovis* in calves challenged with *M bovis* when compared with nonvaccinated, but challenged, controls.[54] A high seroprevalence (60.1%) to BoHV-1 was detected in a yak (*Poephagus grunniens*) farm experiencing an outbreak of abortion and keratoconjunctivitis; no animals had previously been vaccinated against BoHV-1.[55] However, more recent work looking at an outbreak of IBK in a beef herd did not show an association between BoHV-1 status and IBK.[56] A potential mechanism to explain the association of IBR with IBK is that BoHV-1 causes immune depression characterized by inhibition of polymorphonuclear cell migration and cell-mediated cytotoxicity, which could predispose the host to superinfection with bacterial pathogens.[57] BoHV-1 also produces host immunosuppression by inhibiting the production of interferon beta, which may also result in secondary infections in the host.[58]

Other alphaherpesviruses have been associated or experimentally shown to cause infectious keratoconjunctivitis-like lesions in a variety of other ruminant species, including mule deer and semidomesticated reindeer and seem to be the primary cause of these lesions in some of these cases.[59–63]

Malignant Catarrhal Fever

Malignant catarrhal fever (MCF) is caused by 1 of 2 γ-herpesviruses: alcelaphine herpesvirus 1 found in wildebeest and ovine herpesvirus 2 found in sheep, both of which can cause MCF in cattle, bison, deer, pigs, and other ungulates.[64–66] The reservoir hosts are inapparent carriers, but susceptible species show fever, depression, ocular and nasal discharge, diarrhea, and frequently do not survive. Cattle become infected through direct contact with a host or through aerosol exposure.[67] Cattle are considered dead-end hosts that do not transmit the virus to herdmates.[68] Although variable in clinical presentation, a common ocular lesion in MCF cases is corneal edema, which may mimic IBK, although cattle with MCF are systemically sick, which is typically not observed in IBK. Other hallmarks of the disease that preclude IBK include the pattern of ocular opacity, with a fine line that spreads centripetally from the limbus, and the presence of concurrent signs such as persistent high fever, salivation, purulent nasal discharge, and generalized lymph node enlargement.[69] One study of chronic and recovered cattle infected with sheep-associated MCF observed the most obvious clinical sign was bilateral ocular lesions.[70] Severity of corneal edema at the time of diagnosis is not correlated with clinical outcome in cases of MCF; however, cases of MCF that did not survive had no improvement of corneal edema during hospitalization and treatment in a prospective study.[71] Other common clinical signs shared with IBK are blepharospasm, ocular discharge, corneal vascularization, conjunctival hyperemia, and miosis. Corneal ulceration, although uncommon in cases of MCF, does occur.[71,72] Anterior uveitis is a common ocular clinical sign in cases of MCF that is usually absent in cases of IBK.[71] Histologically, MCF ocular lesions are characterized by mitotic figures in lymphoblasts, which is not a finding in IBK lesions.[72]

Listeria monocytogenes

L monocytogenes can cause ocular infections that may resemble IBK, which is characterized by keratoconjunctivitis and uveitis, frequently called "silage eye."[73,74] An excellent review with more detail can be found on this condition.[74] Briefly, Listeria has been shown experimentally to directly penetrate corneal epithelial cells and cause ocular infections, demonstrating that contact of ocular epithelium with concentrated bacteria, potentially through feed, may be a route of entry, thus the common name of silage eye.[75,76] The ability to infect bovine conjunctiva seems in some strains to be associated with resistance to lysozyme.[77] Exposure keratitis secondary to facial nerve palsy caused by infection also seems to be involved.[78] Clinically, ocular infections with L monocytogenes differ from IBK, whereas in the former, the conjunctivitis is nonpurulent, the cornea has minimal changes, and lesions are usually unilateral.[79] Outbreak descriptions involve slow spread over several weeks with an intraherd prevalence that ranged between 7% and 29%.[79] Three out of 170 cases submitted to a diagnostic laboratory were bovine ocular infections with 4 different subtypes isolated.[80,81] Outbreaks have also been associated with baleage-fed animals.[82] L monocytogenes infections in cattle associated with silage may be more complex than initially thought. One study looking at an outbreak of *L monocytogenes* (which primarily caused reproductive infections) in a large system using genomic analysis demonstrated that 3 distinct strains were isolated from animals and only one strain matched those found in silage sources.[83]

Chlamydia spp

Chlamydia spp are nonmotile obligate intracellular bacteria with small genomes that can replicate in a wide variety of host cells.[84] Although the nomenclature of members of this genus has been in flux, there are 10 valid species described, 2 of which infect cattle: *Chlamydia pecorum* and *Chlamydia abortus,* which were previously classified as *Chlamydia psittaci.*[85–88] Infections with *Chlamydia* spp in cattle typically involve mucosal cells or penetration of mucosal surfaces to establish systemic infection, and infectious elementary bodies are shed in feces, nasal, ocular, and reproductive exudates.[89] Diseases in cattle include enteric disease, respiratory disease, polyarthritis-serositis, and sporadic bovine encephalomyelitis.[89] However, asymptomatic infections seem common with one study finding 61% prevalence in normal calves.[90] The age of the calf when exposed in addition to the virulence of the strain seem to have impact on the type and severity of disease observed.[91]

Given the infection of mucosal surfaces, *Chlamydia* spp have long been associated with conjunctivitis in lambs and reindeer among other species, although the relationship with conjunctivitis in cattle is less clear.[92,93] However, it is thought that infections in cattle are likely to resemble other species. Calves experimentally inoculated with *Chlamydia* that resulted in systemic infection and polyarthritis also developed conjunctivitis and subsequent blindness that involved the retina and optic nerve.[94] One report describes 3 outbreaks of IBK-like disease in cattle, one of which lasted 5 months and had morbidity of 100% where the only agent detected was *Chlamydia* sp using PCR.[95] Seven out of 47 conjunctival biopsy samples collected from Kansas cattle with signs consistent with IBK, representing 35 herds, had detectable Chlamydial proteins by enzyme-linked immunosorbent assay.[96] In a study of ruminants in India, 2 out of 8 cattle with clinical keratoconjunctivitis were positive by PCR for *Chlamydia* spp (*C abortus* and *C psittaci*).[97] In another survey, high percentages of both clinical (88%) and nonclinical (68%) cattle were found to be positive for *C psittaci* by PCR in a study conducted in Egypt.[98] A study conducted in India revealed that 3% of ocular infections in cattle with conjunctivitis showed evidence of Chlamydia inclusions in conjunctival smears.[99] Other outbreaks have indicated *C psittaci* detection in association with *M bovis.*[100]

Much remains unclear about the role of *Chlamydia* spp in bovine disease in general, including ocular disease. Diagnosis of chlamydial infections is challenging, and there may be underdiagnosis and underreporting of this pathogen in cattle.[101] However, as methods and technologies advance to detect and sequence these organisms, more is being understood. For example, a specific multilocus sequence type of *C pecorum* (ST23) is associated with ocular infections in sheep and seems to be widespread in livestock including cattle.[102,103] Cattle infected with *Chlamydia* have been reported to have growth reduction; however, they seem to be largely subclinical or nonclincal.[88,90,104,105]

SUMMARY

Although IBK has classically been associated with *Moraxella* organisms, there has been work exploring associations with other pathogenic and opportunistic bacteria and ocular lesions in cattle. Many of these pathogens are extremely challenging to study due to their minimal ability to survive outside of hosts and study in vitro. However, as technological advances progress, tools are becoming available to study them using molecular and next-generation sequencing and other approaches. Additional research needs to be conducted into the association of these challenging microbes, in particular *Myco bovoculi,* and their association and prevalence in both animals with IBK and normal animals.

CLINICS CARE POINTS

- Determination of the cause of outbreaks is challenging, especially when they may involve poorly understood or uncommon pathogens or opportunistic infections with commensals.

- Organisms other than *Moraxella* spp have been implicated as causes of IBK-like clinical disease.

- *Mycoplasma* spp, *Ureaplasma* spp, *Chlamydia* spp, *L monocytogenes*, BoHV-1, and γ-herpesviruses can produce ocular lesions in cattle.

- Syndromic PCR panels that include non-Moraxella agents may help rule out some of the less common etiologic agents.[30]

- Advanced technologies including molecular characterization of potential pathogens and metagenomics tools will help elucidate the roles other agents play in IBK.

DISCLOSURE

The authors have nothing to disclose.

REFERENCES

1. Brown DR, May M, Bradbury JM, et al. Mycoplasma. Bergey's Manual of Systematics of Archaea and Bacteria 2018:1-78.
2. Nicholas R, R.D A, McAuliffe L. Mycoplasma Diseases of Ruminants. Mycoplasma Diseases of Ruminants 2008:1-239.
3. Nicola I, Cerutti F, Grego E, et al. Characterization of the upper and lower respiratory tract microbiota in Piedmontese calves. Microbiome 2017;5(1):152.
4. Timsit E, Workentine M, Schryvers AB, et al. Evolution of the nasopharyngeal microbiota of beef cattle from weaning to 40 days after arrival at a feedlot. Vet Microbiol 2016;187:75–81.
5. McMullen C, Orsel K, Alexander TW, et al. Evolution of the nasopharyngeal bacterial microbiota of beef calves from spring processing to 40 days after feedlot arrival. Vet Microbiol 2018;225:139–48.
6. Lima SF, Teixeira AGV, Higgins CH, et al. The upper respiratory tract microbiome and its potential role in bovine respiratory disease and otitis media. Scientific Rep 2016;6(1):29050.
7. Cullen JN, Lithio A, Seetharam AS, et al. Microbial community sequencing analysis of the calf eye microbiota and relationship to infectious bovine keratoconjunctivitis. Vet Microbiol 2017;207:267–79.
8. De Rudder C, Arroyo MC, Lebeer S, et al. Dual and Triple Epithelial Coculture Model Systems with Donor-Derived Microbiota and THP-1 macrophages to mimic host-microbe interactions in the human sinonasal cavities. MSPHERE 2020;5(1). e00916-19.
9. Bartenslager AC, Althuge ND, Loy JD, et al. Longitudinal assessment of the bovine ocular bacterial community dynamics in calves. Anim Microbiome 2021;3(1):16.

10. Dudek K, Nicholas RAJ, Szacawa E, et al. Mycoplasma bovis infections—occurrence, diagnosis and control. Pathogens 2020;9(8).

11. Langford EV, Leach RH. Characterization of a mycoplasma isolated from infectious bovine keratoconjunctivitis: M. bovoculi sp. nov. Can J Microbiol 1973; 19(11):1435–44.

12. Langford EV, Dorward WJ. A mycoplasma isolated from cattle with infectious bovine keratoconjunctivitis. Can J Comp Med 1969;33(4):275–9.

13. Barber DM, Jones GE, Wood A. Microbial flora of the eyes of cattle. Vet Rec 1986;118(8):204–6.

14. Salih BA, Rosenbusch RF. Attachment of Mycoplasma bovoculi to bovine conjunctival epithelium and lung fibroblasts. Am J Vet Res 1988;49(10):1661–4.

15. Rosenbusch RF. Bovine pinkeye: etiology and pathogenesis. Bovine Pract 1985; 1985(20):150–2.

16. Calcutt MJ, Foecking MF. Complete Genome Sequence of Mycoplasma bovoculi Strain M165/69T (ATCC 29104). Genome announcements 2014;2(1). e00115-00114.

17. Yogev D, Rosengarten R, Watson-McKown R, et al. Molecular basis of Mycoplasma surface antigenic variation: a novel set of divergent genes undergo spontaneous mutation of periodic coding regions and 5' regulatory sequences. EMBO J 1991;10(13):4069–79.

18. Rosenbusch RF, Knudtson WU. Bovine mycoplasmal conjunctivitis: experimental reproduction and characterization of the disease. The Cornell veterinarian 1980;70(4):307–20.

19. Nayar PS, Saunders JR. Infectious bovine keratoconjunctivitis I. Experimental production. Can J Comp Med 1975;39(1):22–31.

20. Friis NF, Pedersen KB. Isolation of Mycoplasma bovoculi from cases of infectious bovine keratoconjunctivitis. Acta Vet Scand 1979;20(1):51–9.

21. Rosenbusch RF. Influence of mycoplasma preinfection on the expression of Moraxella bovis pathogenicity. Am J Vet Res 1983;44(9):1621–4.

22. Rosenbusch RF, Ostle AG. Mycoplasma bovoculi infection increases ocular colonization by Moraxella ovis in calves. Am J Vet Res 1986;47(6):1214–6.

23. Salih BA, Rosenbusch RF. Antibody response in calves experimentally or naturally exposed to Mycoplasma bovoculi. Vet Microbiol 1986;11(1–2):93–102.

24. Salih BA, Ostle AG, Rosenbusch RF. Vaccination of cattle with Mycoplasma bovoculi antigens: evidence for field immunity. Comp Immunol Microbiol Infect Dis 1987;10(2):109–16.

25. Salih BA, Rosenbusch RF. Identification and localization of a 94 kDa membrane protein found in Mycoplasma bovoculi strains. Comp Immunol Microbiol Infect Dis 1998;21(4):281–90.

26. Salih BA, Rosenbusch RF. Cross-reactive proteins among eight bovine mycoplasmas detected by monoclonal antibodies. Comp Immunol Microbiol Infect Dis 2001;24(2):103–11.

27. Norian LA, Rosenbusch RF. Mycoplasma bovoculi–augmented bovine natural killer activity. Comp Immunol Microbiol Infect Dis 1993;16(2):113–22.

28. Bansal VK, Garg DN, Singh Y. Seroprevalence of Mycoplasma bovoculi antibodies by ELISA in conjunctivitis affected and healthy bovines. Haryana Veterinarian 2002;41:33–7.

29. Schnee C, Heller M, Schubert E, et al. Point prevalence of infection with Mycoplasma bovoculi and Moraxella spp. in cattle at different stages of infectious bovine keratoconjunctivitis. Vet J 2015;203(1):92–6.

30. Zheng W, Porter E, Noll L, et al. A multiplex real-time PCR assay for the detection and differentiation of five bovine pinkeye pathogens. J Microbiol Methods 2019; 160:87–92.
31. Burki S, Frey J, Pilo P. Virulence, persistence and dissemination of Mycoplasma bovis. Vet Microbiol 2015;179(1–2):15–22.
32. Ayling RD, Bashiruddin SE, Nicholas RAJ. Mycoplasma species and related organisms isolated from ruminants in Britain between 1990 and 2000. Vet Rec 2004;155(14):413–6.
33. Dando SJ, Sweeney EL, Knox CL. Ureaplasma. Bergey's Manual of Systematics of Archaea and Bacteria 2019:1-28.
34. Alberti A, Addis MF, Chessa B, et al. Molecular and antigenic characterization of a mycoplasma bovis strain causing an outbreak of infectious keratoconjunctivitis. J Vet Diagn Invest 2006;18(1):41–51.
35. Jack EJ, Moring J, Boughton E. Isolation of Mycoplasma bovis from an outbreak of infectious bovine kerato conjunctivitis. Vet Rec 1977;101(14):287.
36. Kirby FD, Nicholas RA. Isolation of Mycoplasma bovis from bullocks' eyes. Vet Rec 1996;138(22):552.
37. Levisohn S, Garazi S, Gerchman I, et al. Diagnosis of a mixed mycoplasma infection associated with a severe outbreak of bovine pinkeye in young calves. J Vet Diagn Invest 2004;16(6):579–81.
38. Naglic T, Sankovic F, Madic J, et al. Mycoplasmas associated with bovine conjunctivitis and keratoconjunctivitis. Acta Vet Hung 1996;44(1):21–4.
39. Pugh GW, Hughes DE, Schulz VD. Infectious bovine keratoconjunctivitis: experimental induction of infection in calves with mycoplasmas and Moraxella bovis. Am J Vet Res 1976;37(5):493–5.
40. HOWARD CJ, GOURLAY RN. Proposal for a Second Species Within the Genus Ureaplasma, Ureaplasma diversum sp. nov. Int J Syst Evol Microbiol 1982;32(4): 446–52.
41. Ross RF. Mycoplasma — Animal Pathogens. In: Kahane I, Adoni A, editors. Rapid diagnosis of mycoplasmas. Boston,: Springer US; 1993. p. 69–109.
42. Gourlay RN, Thomas LH. The isolation of large colony and T-strain mycoplasmas from cases of bovine kerato-conjunctivitis. Vet Rec 1969;84(16):416–7.
43. Crane MB, Hughes CA. Can Ureaplasma diversum be transmitted from donor to recipient through the embryo? Two case reports outlining U. diversum losses in bovine embryo pregnancies. Can Vet J 2018;59(1):43–6.
44. Truscott RB. Nongenital mycoplasma infections in cattle. Can Vet J 1981;22(11): 335–8.
45. Abinanti FR, Plumer GJ. The isolation of infectious bovine rhinotracheitis virus from cattle affected with conjunctivitis-observations on the experimental infection. Am J Vet Res 1961;22:13–7.
46. Al-Bana AS, Majeed AK, Barhoom S. Isolation of infectious bovine rhinotracheitis virus from calves affected with keratoconjunctivitis. Iraqi J Vet Sci 1998;11(2): 227–31.
47. Bartha A, Magdalena J, Liebermann H, et al. Isolation and properties of a bovine herpes virus from a calf with respiratory disease and keratoconjunctivitis. Arch Exp Veterinarmed 1967;21(2):615–23.
48. Hughes JP, Olander HJ, Wada M. Keratoconjuctivitis associated with infectious bovine rhinotracheitis. J Am Vet Med Assoc 1964;145:32–9.
49. Sykes JA, Dmochowski L, Grey CE, et al. Isolation of a virus from infectious bovine kerato-conjunctivitis. Proc Soc Exp Biol Med Soc Exp Biol Med 1962; 111:51–7.

50. St G TD. Keratoconjunctivitis associated with infectious bovine rhinotracheitis infection in Victorian cattle. Aust Vet J 1965;41:222–3.
51. Mohanty SB, Lillie MG. Relationship of infectious bovine keratoconjunctivitis virus to the virus of infectious bovine rhinotracheitis. The Cornell veterinarian 1970;60(1):3–9.
52. Schulze P, Liebermann H, Hantschel H, et al. Light and electron microscopical examinations of a new bovine herpes virus. Russ Engl Sum Arch Exp Veterinarmed 1967;21(3):747–59.
53. Pugh GW Jr, Hughes DE, Packer RA. Bovine infectious keratoconjunctivitis: interactions of Moraxella bovis and infectious bovine rhinotracheitis virus. Am J Vet Res 1970;31(4):653–62.
54. George LW, Ardans A, Mihalyi J, et al. Enhancement of infectious bovine keratoconjunctivitis by modified-live infectious bovine rhinotracheitis virus vaccine. Am J Vet Res 1988;49(11):1800–6.
55. Nandi S, Kumar M. Serological evidence of bovine herpesvirus-1 (BoHV-1) infection in yaks (Peophagus grunniens) from the National Research Centre on Yak, India. Trop Anim Health Prod 2010;42(6):1041–2.
56. Zbrun MV, Zielinski GC, Piscitelli HC, et al. Dynamics of Moraxella bovis infection and humoral immune response to bovine herpes virus type 1 during a natural outbreak of infectious bovine keratoconjunctivitis in beef calves. J Vet Sci 2011;12(4):347–52.
57. Wyler R, Engels M, Schwyzer M. Infectious Bovine Rhinotracheitis/Vulvovaginitis (BHV1). In: Wittmann G, editor. Herpesvirus diseases of cattle, horses, and pigs. Boston: Springer US; 1989. p. 1–72.
58. da Silva LF, Sinani D, Jones C. ICP27 protein encoded by bovine herpesvirus type 1 (bICP27) interferes with promoter activity of the bovine genes encoding beta interferon 1 (IFN-β1) and IFN-β3. Virus Res 2012;169(1):162–8.
59. Tryland M, Romano JS, Marcin N, et al. Cervid herpesvirus 2 and not Moraxella bovoculi caused keratoconjunctivitis in experimentally inoculated semi-domesticated Eurasian tundra reindeer. Acta veterinaria Scand 2017;59(1):23.
60. Muñoz Gutiérrez JF, Sondgeroth KS, Williams ES, et al. Infectious keratoconjunctivitis in free-ranging mule deer in Wyoming: a retrospective study and identification of a novel alphaherpesvirus. J Vet Diagn Invest 2018;30(5):663–70.
61. Sánchez Romano J, Mørk T, Laaksonen S, et al. Infectious keratoconjunctivitis in semi-domesticated Eurasian tundra reindeer (Rangifer tarandus tarandus): microbiological study of clinically affected and unaffected animals with special reference to cervid herpesvirus 2. BMC Vet Res 2018;14(1):15.
62. Tryland M, Das Neves CG, Sunde M, et al. Cervid Herpesvirus 2, the primary agent in an outbreak of infectious keratoconjunctivitis in semidomesticated reindeer. J Clin Microbiol 2009;47(11):3707–13.
63. Sánchez Romano J, Sørensen KK, Larsen AK, et al. Ocular Histopathological Findings in Semi-Domesticated Eurasian Tundra Reindeer (Rangifer tarandus tarandus) with Infectious Keratoconjunctivitis after Experimental Inoculation with Cervid Herpesvirus 2. Viruses 2020;12(9):1007.
64. Loken T, Aleksandersen M, Reid H, et al. Malignant catarrhal fever caused by ovine herpesvirus-2 in pigs in Norway. Vet Rec 1998;143(17):464–7.
65. Reid HW, Buxton D, Berrie E, et al. Malignant catarrhal fever. Vet Rec 1984; 114(24):581–3.
66. Schultheiss PC, Collins JK, Spraker TR, et al. Epizootic malignant catarrhal fever in three bison herds: differences from cattle and association with ovine herpesvirus-2. J Vet Diagn Invest 2000;12(6):497–502.

67. Russell GC, Stewart JP, Haig DM. Malignant catarrhal fever: a review. Vet J 2009;179(3):324–35.
68. Mushi EZ, Rurangirwa FR. Malignant catarrhal fever virus shedding by infected cattle. Bull Anim Health Prod Afr 1981;29(1):111–2.
69. Crawford TB, O'Toole D, Li H. Malignant Catarrhal Fever. In: Howard JL, Smith RA, editors. Current veterinary therapy 4: food animal practice. Philadephipa: Saunders; 1999. p. 306–9.
70. O'Toole D, Li H, Miller D, et al. Chronic and recovered cases of sheep-associated malignant catarrhal fever in cattle. Vet Rec 1997;140(20):519.
71. Zemljic T, Pot SA, Haessig M, et al. Clinical ocular findings in cows with malignant catarrhal fever: ocular disease progression and outcome in 25 cases (2007-2010). Vet Ophthalmol 2012;15(1):46–52.
72. Whiteley HE, Young S, Liggitt HD, et al. Ocular lesions of bovine malignant catarrhal fever. Vet Pathol 1985;22(3):219–25.
73. Kummeneje K, Mikkelsen T. Isolation of Listeria monocytogenes type 04 from cases of keratoconjunctivitis in cattle and sheep. Nord Vet Med 1975;27(3):144–9.
74. Erdogan HM. Listerial Keratoconjunctivitis and Uveitis (Silage Eye). Vet Clin North Am Food Anim Pract 2010;26(3):505–10.
75. Racz P, Tenner K, Szivessy K. Electron microscopic studies in experimental keratoconjunctivitis listeriosa. I. Penetration of Listeria monocytogenes into corneal epithelial cells. Acta Microbiol Acad Sci Hung 1970;17(3):221–36.
76. Stams A. [Studies in cases of experimental eye infections with Listeria monocytogenes]. Albrecht Von Graefes Arch Klin Exp Ophthalmol 1967;173(1):1–20.
77. Warren J, Owen AR, Glanvill A, et al. A new bovine conjunctiva model shows that Listeria monocytogenes invasion is associated with lysozyme resistance. Vet Microbiol 2015;179(1):76–81.
78. Rebhun WC, deLahunta A. Diagnosis and treatment of bovine listeriosis. J Am Vet Med Assoc 1982;180(4):395–8.
79. Morgan JH. Infectious keratoconjunctivitis in cattle associated with Listeria monocytocytogenes. Vet Rec 1977;100(6):113–4.
80. Evans K, Smith M, McDonough P, et al. Eye Infections due to Listeria Monocytogenes in Three Cows and One Horse. J Vet Diagn Invest 2004;16(5):464–9.
81. Low JC, Donachie W. A review of Listeria monocytogenes and listeriosis. Vet J 1997;153(1):9–29.
82. Laven RA, Lawrence KR. An outbreak of iritis and uveitis in dairy cattle at pasture associated with the supplementary feeding of baleage. New Zealand Vet J 2006;54(3):151–2.
83. Whitman KJ, Bono JL, Clawson ML, et al. Genomic-based identification of environmental and clinical Listeria monocytogenes strains associated with an abortion outbreak in beef heifers. BMC Vet Res 2020;16(1):70.
84. Horn M. Chlamydiae. Bergey's Manual of Systematics of Archaea and Bacteria 2015:1-2.
85. Sachse K, Bavoil PM, Kaltenboeck B, et al. Emendation of the family Chlamydiaceae: proposal of a single genus, Chlamydia, to include all currently recognized species. Syst Appl Microbiol 2015;38(2):99–103.
86. Fukushi H, Hirai K. Proposal of Chlamydia pecorum sp. nov. for Chlamydia strains derived from ruminants. Int J Syst Bacteriol 1992;42(2):306–8.
87. Parte AC, Sardà Carbasse J, Meier-Kolthoff JP, et al. List of Prokaryotic names with Standing in Nomenclature (LPSN) moves to the DSMZ. Int J Syst Evol Microbiol 2020;70(11):5607–12.

88. Poudel A, Elsasser TH, Rahman Kh S, et al. Asymptomatic endemic Chlamydia pecorum infections reduce growth rates in calves by up to 48 percent. PLoS One 2012;7(9):e44961.
89. Perez-Martinez JA, Storz J. Chamydial infections in cattle- Part 1. Mod Vet Pract 1985;66(8):517–22.
90. Jee J, Degraves FJ, Kim T, et al. High prevalence of natural Chlamydophila species infection in calves. J Clin Microbiol 2004;42(12):5664–72.
91. Storz J, Eugster AK, Altera KP, et al. Behavior of different bovine chlamydial agents in newborn calves. J Comp Pathol 1971;81(2):299–307.
92. Hopkins JB, Stephenson EH, Storz J, et al. Conjunctivitis associated with chlamydial polyarthritis in lambs. J Am Vet Med Assoc 1973;163(10):1157–60.
93. Romano JS, Leijon M, Hagstrom A, et al. Chlamydia pecorum associated with an outbreak of infectious keratoconjunctivitis in semi-domesticated reindeer in Sweden. Front In Vet Sci 2019;6:14.
94. Storz J. Overview of Animal Diseases Induced by Chlamydial Infections. In: Barron A, editor. Microbiology of Chlamydia, vol. 1. Boca Raton: CRC Press; 1988. p. 264.
95. Otter A, Twomey DF, Rowe NS, et al. Suspected chlamydial keratoconjunctivitis in British cattle. Vet Rec 2003;152(25):787–8.
96. Daniels EK, Cole DE. Chlamydial proteins found in bovine conjunctival biopsies. Bovine Pract 1991;(26):142.
97. Gupta S, Chahota R, Bhardwaj B, et al. Identification of chlamydiae and mycoplasma species in ruminants with ocular infections. Lett Appl Microbiol 2015; 60(2):135–9.
98. Osman KM, Ali HA, ElJakee JA, et al. Prevalence of chlamydophila psittaci infections in the eyes of cattle, buffaloes, sheep and goats in contact with a human population. Transboundary Emerging Dis 2013;60(3):245–51.
99. Samantaray SS, Das PK, Das RK, et al. Cytological and microbiological evaluation of conjunctivitis in cattle. Indian J Vet Med 1995;15(2):79–83.
100. Batta MK, Sharma M, Joshi VB, et al. Infectious bovine keratoconjunctivitis in a dairy farm: Etiologic investigations. Indian Vet J 1996;73(7):713–7.
101. Walker E, Lee EJ, Timms P, et al. Chlamydia pecorum infections in sheep and cattle: A common and under-recognised infectious disease with significant impact on animal health. Vet J 2015;206(3):252–60.
102. Jelocnik M, Frentiu FD, Timms P, et al. Multilocus Sequence Analysis Provides Insights into Molecular Epidemiology of Chlamydia pecorum Infections in Australian Sheep, Cattle, and Koalas. J Clin Microbiol 2013;51(8):2625.
103. Jelocnik M, Walker E, Pannekoek Y, et al. Evaluation of the relationship between Chlamydia pecorum sequence types and disease using a species-specific multi-locus sequence typing scheme (MLST). Vet Microbiol 2014;174(1): 214–22.
104. Reinhold P, Sachse K, Kaltenboeck B. Chlamydiaceae in cattle: Commensals, trigger organisms, or pathogens? Vet J 2011;189(3):257–67.
105. Walker E, Moore C, Shearer P, et al. Clinical, diagnostic and pathologic features of presumptive cases of Chlamydia pecorum-associated arthritis in Australian sheep flocks. BMC Vet Res 2016;12:193.

The Role of Environmental Factors in the Epidemiology of Infectious Bovine Keratoconjunctivitis

Gabriele Maier, DVM, MPVM, PhD, DACVPM[a],*, Binh Doan, BS[b],
Annette M. O'Connor, BVSc, MVSc, DVSc, FANZCVS[c]

KEYWORDS

- Infectious bovine keratoconjunctivitis • Environment • Face flies
- *Musca autumnalis* De Geer • Ultraviolet radiation • Plant awns

KEY POINTS

- Face flies have close associations in space and time with cattle eyes and the occurrence of infectious bovine keratoconjunctivitis (IBK).
- Laboratory studies have shown face flies to be capable of transmitting *Moraxella bovis* between cattle eyes, resulting in IBK. Field studies have not been able to show that prevalence of *M bovis* on face flies is associated with incidence of IBK. No other IBK pathogens have been studied in association with face flies.
- Face fly control seems to be associated with reduced incidence of IBK, but the magnitude of control that can be expected is unclear due to small studies.
- Ultraviolet radiation causes bovine corneal irritation and increased number of corneal dark cells. *M bovis* preferentially attaches to corneal dark cells, which are mostly devoid of microscopic surface projections.
- Mechanical irritation or ocular foreign bodies in the form of grass awns or dust can mimic signs of IBK or predispose to IBK.

INTRODUCTION

Infectious bovine keratoconjunctivitis (IBK) is a multifactorial ocular disease of cattle. The gram-negative bacterium *Moraxella bovis* (*M bovis*) is the infectious agent most

[a] Department of Population Health and Reproduction, School of Veterinary Medicine, Davis, 1 Shields Avenue, VM3B, Davis, CA 95616, USA; [b] Carver College of Medicine, University of Iowa, 51 Newton Road, 1-400 BSB, Iowa City, IA 52242, USA; [c] Department of Large Animal Clinical Sciences, College of Veterinary Medicine, Michigan State University, 784 Wilson Road, Room G-100, East Lansing, MI 48824, USA
* Corresponding author.
E-mail address: gumaier@ucdavis.edu

Vet Clin Food Anim 37 (2021) 309–320
https://doi.org/10.1016/j.cvfa.2021.03.006
0749-0720/21/© 2021 Elsevier Inc. All rights reserved.
vetfood.theclinics.com

frequently associated with the disease. Environmental factors such as the mechanical vector *Musca autumnalis* De Geer, ultraviolet (UV) radiation, or mechanical irritation of the cornea from plants or dust are thought to contribute to the pathology of IBK. The only pathogen that has been studied in relation to face flies as mechanical vectors is *M bovis*. Information on transmission by face flies of other potential IBK pathogens is missing so far. The available evidence for the contribution of environmental factors to IBK is discussed in this article.

FACE FLIES

The most researched environmental factor implicated in the cause of IBK is the face fly, *M autumnalis* De Geer (**Fig. 1**), although most of the research was conducted between 50 and 20 years ago. The putative role of the face fly in the epidemiology of IBK has been as a mechanical vector for the bacterial pathogen *M bovis* and as a source of corneal injury through its feeding activity on ocular secretions. As one of only 2 species of the genus *Musca* in North America, the face fly was first reported in North America in 1952[1] and has since spread throughout the United States and temperate regions of Canada.[2] The face fly is suspected to have been accidently introduced into North America in the 1940s, a proposition that is supported by the species' absence from insect collections in museums before 1952. Face flies reproduce continuously during the summer months when their eggs and larvae develop in fresh cow manure. In the fall, triggered by a shortening photoperiod, nulliparous flies seek out a hibernaculum and spend the winter in prereproductive diapause until they start reproducing in the spring.[3] Its distribution, life cycle, and close association with cattle eyes explain why *M autumnalis* De Geer has been an obvious target for investigation as a risk factor for IBK. Determining the extent to which face flies are a causal component of the epidemiology is difficult because of the challenges in differentiating association and correlation from causation. To this end, it has been proposed that to qualify as an arthropod vector for a specific pathogen the following 5 criteria should be considered, which are discussed in the following section.[4]

Demonstration of Feeding or Effective Contact with the Host Under Natural Conditions

Face flies spend various amounts of time on cattle eyes; one study reported that less than 4% of the face fly population can be found on cattle at any one time.[5] Females

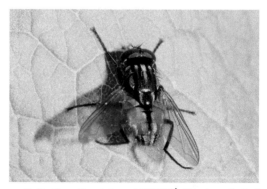

Fig. 1. *Musca autumnalis* De Geer Dominique MARTIRÉ. The face fly is similar in appearance to the house fly, averages 7 to 8 mm in length, and the thorax displays 4 dark stripes.

commonly feed on bodily fluids including tears.[6,7] Mean face fly visits on cattle eyes last 42 seconds with many only lasting a second and the longest stays lasting more than 3 minutes.[8] Eyes affected by IBK have longer mean staying times of 105 seconds possibly due to the increased lacrimation and higher abundance of nutrients for face flies, which supports a mechanism for the face fly's role in the transmission of bacteria from one eye to another.[8] Exposure of cattle to *M bovis*–free face flies in a laboratory setting caused lacrimation and microscopic conjunctival and corneal damage.[9] Rasping with their prestomal teeth,[10] featuring jagged and sharp terminal points[11] that can penetrate the corneal epithelium 30 to 40 μm thick during feeding on conjunctiva, causes mechanical irritation by *M autumnalis* De Geer (**Fig. 2**).

A Biological Association in Time and Space of the Suspected Arthropod Species and Occurrence of Infection in the Host

There are spatial and temporal correlations between the abundance and distribution of the face fly and the incidence of IBK. Face flies are most active at temperatures between 25°C and 29°C (77–84°F), and face fly populations in North America peak in late May, late June, and early August,[6] correlating with seasons when IBK is most prevalent. The arthropod feeds on cattle eye secretions and is often found on the face and around the eyes of cattle. Face flies' occurrence on cattle has diurnal patterns with highest numbers observed when cattle are resting in the shade, and air temperature, relative humidity, and wind speed do not affect these daily patterns.[12]

However, on a larger temporal scale, the association is less clear. IBK was already a known cattle disease in the United States before introduction of the face fly, although reports of the face fly's spread through North America were accompanied by complaints of increasing incidence of cattle eye disorders.[13] Likewise, the geographic distribution of the face fly, which includes the temperate latitudes of Europe, northern Africa, and central Asia as well as North America[2] does overlap but not completely coincide with regions where cattle suffer from IBK. The face fly, therefore, may be a contributing factor but does not seem to be a necessary factor for the transmission of IBK.

Demonstration that the Arthropod, Under Natural Conditions, Harbors the Infective Agent in the Infective Stage

There is observational evidence that flies can be infected with *M bovis*. Several studies have documented recovery of *M bovis* from face flies. However, only a small percentage (0.6%–4.1%) of face flies that were caught in close proximity to cattle herds with IBK cases were culture positive for *M bovis*.[14] The infective stage criterion is not relevant to bacteria such as *M bovis* and is more applicable to pathogens with lifecycles such as Plasmodium spp. More relevant to bacteria is the ability to document transmission by the vector to other surfaces. Some research has documented that naturally infected flies can transmit *M bovis* to other surfaces, that is, agar.[15]

The Ability of the Arthropod to Transfer the Infectious Agent Under Controlled Conditions

In laboratory settings, face flies have shown to be able to transmit *M bovis* from cell culture preparations to sterile culture plates for at least 6 hours after exposure[16] as well as from pure cultures to cattle eyes.[17] Arends and colleagues (1984) were also able to document 7 cases of IBK in 16 calves exposed to flies infected with *M bovis*, compared with 0 cases in the 16 calves exposed to flies without *M bovis* (**Fig. 3**).[17]

Viable *M bovis* can be recovered from the crop and midgut of face flies for up to 48 hours after feeding on a trypticase-soy broth suspension of *M bovis* under laboratory conditions.[18] *M bovis* is also recovered in the crops of face flies feeding on cattle

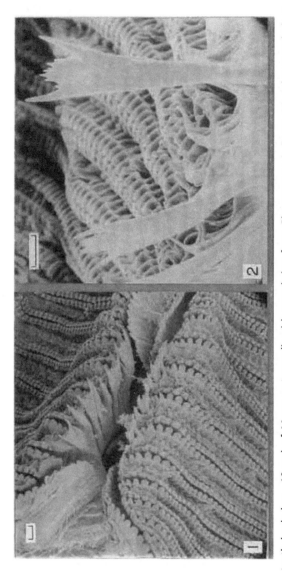

Fig. 2. Prestomal teeth (scale bar—10 μm) of *Musca autumnalis* with permission from Giangaspero A, Broce AB. Micromorphology of the prestomal teeth and feeding behaviour of Musca autumnalis, M.larvipara and M.osiris (Diptera: Muscidae). Med Vet Entomol. 1993;7(4):398-400.

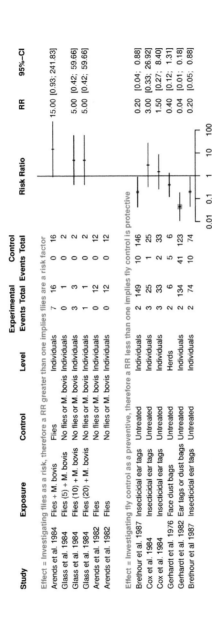

Fig. 3. Forest plot of the risk ratio reported for experimental and field studies that evaluated either flies as a risk factor for the occurrence of Infectios Bovine Keratoconjunctivitis or fly control products as a protective intervention.

eyes in various stages of IBK—most frequently from convalescent cases and to a lesser extent from more acute cases. One reason could be that cattle tend to keep their eyes shut during the acute phase of IBK, which lessens opportunity for exposure to flies.[19] Face flies regurgitate *M bovis* while feeding on eye secretions and their proboscis touches the surface of the cornea. At least 10 flies per eye were required for successful transmission of *M bovis* to cattle corneas resulting in IBK, at least under laboratory conditions.[20]

A Correlation Between Vector Population Levels and Disease Incidence in Susceptible Hosts

Several investigators have attempted to evaluate either correlation or associations between flies and IBK lesions at the individual cow level and at the herd level. These correlations or associations should be separated into associations between fly numbers and IBK and associations between fly numbers with *M bovis* and IBK, as these represent different lines of investigation (**Fig. 4**). These correlations can further be separated into experimental and observational. An early observational study conducted between 1963 and 1965 that recorded numbers of flies on cows' faces and incidence of IBK found a weak positive correlation between those factors.[21] A similar weak positive

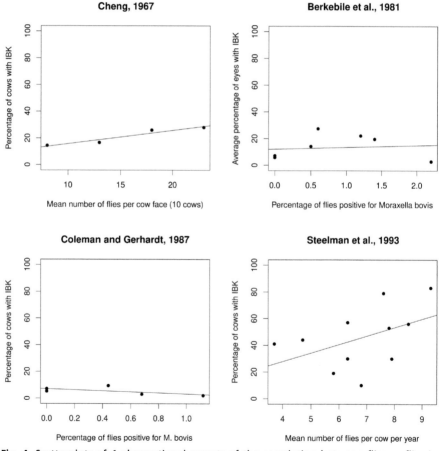

Fig. 4. Scatterplots of 4 observational reports of the correlation between flies or flies infected with *Moraxella bovis* and Infectious Bovine Keratoconjunctivitis lesions.

correlation between fly numbers and IBK was observed by others[22] (see **Fig. 4**). In experimental infection studies, the numbers of study animals are too small to make any inference that exposure to more flies can induce IBK in calves (see **Fig. 3**). The incidence of IBK has also been observed to be decreased in cattle after fly control products are applied in 2 of 3 studies, supporting a causal role for face flies in IBK[15,23,24] (see **Fig. 3**). The agent used for fly control is important, and not all external parasite control agents are equally effective in controlling this insect. Insecticide-impregnated ear tags containing cypermethrin, fenvalerate, or flucythrinate, all belonging to the pyrethroid insecticides, led to greater than 90% reduction in fly numbers observed on cattle, and resulted in fewer pinkeye cases in the cypermethrin-treated herds compared with control, that is, 1 case in the cypermethrin-treated herds and 9 IBK cases in untreated herds; however the herd sizes were not reported. The flucythrinate trial had only 1 case of IBK in the treated cattle and 0 in the control herd, and no IBK occurred in the fenvalerate trials in either the treated or control herds.[25]

Whether ear tags or a pour-on formulation of cypermethrin is used does not seem to affect IBK incidence.[26] Injectable extended-release eprinomectin resulted in fewer pinkeye cases in cows (8.4% vs 4.6%, $P = .06$) compared with injectable doramectin, without an observed reduction in fly burden and although extended-release eprinomectin is not labeled for fly control.[27] There was no observed difference in IBK in calves, although the data were not reported ($P = .43$). However, both of these studies did not include a negative control, so the true impact on IBK incidence cannot be inferred from the results.

Fly control is a preventive measure that should be incorporated into an IBK control plan; however, judicious use of insecticides must be stressed.[28] Although no reports on problems of face fly resistance to insecticides exist, perhaps because of the large refugia of face fly populations, repetitive use of the same class of chemical or prolonged exposure to sublethal doses of a chemical has led to insecticide resistance in other ectoparasite species.[29,30] Integrated pest management including chemical and nonchemical pest reduction measures may prolong the usefulness of available drugs.[31,32] Removal of insecticide-impregnated ear tags at the end of the fly season or at the end of the active duration determined by the manufacturer as well as rotation of different classes of insecticides are part of a judicious ectoparasite control program. An excellent resource for choosing pesticides in livestock species is the database for control of insect pests of animals (https://www.veterinaryentomology.org/vetpestx).[33]

Interestingly, in observational studies there is little evidence that the burden of infection of face flies with M bovis and IBK levels are correlated (see **Fig. 4**).[14,34] Gerhardt and colleagues (1982) reported that M bovis is more frequently cultured from face flies in herds or groups of cattle with higher incidence of IBK.[15] However, there is the potential for information bias to explain the observed result. The study was an assessment of insecticides aimed at affecting IBK by reducing fly numbers in 6 untreated herds and 6 treated herds (those results are presented in **Fig. 3**). The investigators used more intensive sampling for M bovis flies in untreated herds (4 positive pools from 45 fly pools) compared with treated herds (0 positive pools from 20 fly pools), resulting in different sensitivity of detection of M bovis–infected flies in the untreated herds compared with the treated herds. Oversampling is a potentially more sensible explanation for the increased detection of more M bovis–infected flies in the untreated herds compared with none in the treated herds. From a biological point of view, it is unclear why insecticide use would differentially reduce the number of flies infected with M bovis. These studies combined might suggest that scarification due to flies is a more likely role in IBK than M bovis transmission due to flies.

ULTRAVIOLET LIGHT

IBK is seasonal in nature, with most cases occurring in the summer months. UV radiation has been recognized as a way to enhance the effect of experimental infections with *M bovis* and to more consistently produce IBK in study animals than by instillation of pathogen onto the eye alone.[35–37] UV radiation has therefore been recognized as a risk factor for the disease and is frequently mentioned in review papers as a contributing factor to the pathology of IBK.[38–40] Maximal solar UV radiation preceded clinical cases of infection with *M bovis* in a beef herd observed over a 5-year period. Exposure of cattle eyes to artificial UV radiation with a sunlamp set at wavelengths to replicate the midsummer sun at noon (280–320 nm) caused severe clinical signs of IBK in combination with *M bovis* infection.[35] Infection with *M bovis* alone or blocking the sunlamp with glass failed to produce the same clinical signs. However, infection in the absence of injurious UV radiation has also been observed.[41]

Exposure to UV radiation is known to cause photokeratitis in the mammalian eye at certain wavelengths and energy, resulting in photophobia and lacrimation.[42,43] Histologically, there is superficial epithelial cell necrosis and destruction of lysosomal membranes in deeper epithelial layers.[44]

Corneal epithelial cells can be categorized as dark, intermediate, or light in their microscopic appearance. Light cells lose the surface projections microvilli and microplicae (ridges) over time and become intermediate and then dark cells.[45,46] The corneas of calves irradiated with UV light seem to have higher numbers of dark cells, prominent round nuclei, and cells in stages of cytoplasmic degeneration.[43] *M bovis* adheres preferentially to bovine corneal dark cells in vitro[43,46–48] as well as in vivo[41] where it is observed in pits that are suspected to result from bacterial contact **(Fig. 5)**.[46] Radiation damage is therefore thought to increase susceptibility of the corneal epithelium to infection with *M bovis* by increasing the number of dark cells, creating epithelial defects, and increasing the cell turnover rate.[43] A hypothesis for the preferential adhesion of *M bovis* to dark cells is that the diminished surface projections in dark cells may expose receptors for *M bovis* adhesins.[41]

Biochemical changes in isolates of *M bovis* cultured during different times of the year have also been observed where hemolysis, agar corrosion, gelatin liquefaction,

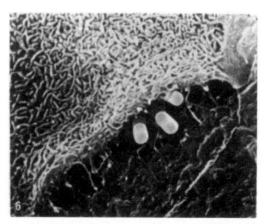

Fig. 5. Moraxella bovis lodged in a space between a light cell showing microplicae and a dark cell, scanning electron microscope image (x 3750). (With permission from Chandler et al. Scanning electron microscope studies on preparations of bovine cornea exposed to *Moraxella bovis*. J. Comp. Path. 1983, Vol 93.)

and litmus milk peptonization occurs more frequently during times of higher energy UV radiation as well as a change from smooth to rough colony type that indicates pili expression.[49]

PLANT AWNS

Irritation from plant awns while grazing or feeding on haylage can cause corneal irritation predisposing to IBK or result in ocular foreign bodies and clinical presentations mimicking IBK.[39,50] However, as we tend to think of IBK as a herd-level diagnosis with a substantial proportion of cattle affected, individual cases of ocular lesions due to plant awns would not constitute IBK. It is speculated, but no data are available, that some pasture plants cause irritation to a large proportion of the herd, and this mechanical trauma is the initiating event that allows *M bovis* to cause ocular lesions. Although it is recommended in some review articles that chemical weed control or cutting fields before irritating weeds go to seed are ways to control unwanted species,[51] there is no evidence of weed control being associated with reduced IBK or high levels of weeds being associated with high levels of IBK.

CLINICS CARE POINTS

- Face fly control should be part of a herd health plan in herds where IBK is a problem. Not all insecticides that target ectoparasites are effective in controlling face flies, so care must be taken when choosing an agent.
- Rotating fly tag chemicals and removing tags at the end of the fly season are part of judicious insecticide use.
- In regions with intense UV radiation, cattle may benefit from available shade to reduce the incidence of IBK.
- Where frequent ocular foreign bodies or irregularly shaped corneal ulcers atypical of IBK are observed in cattle, feedstuffs should be inspected for possible sources. Chemical weed control or cutting of fields before irritating weeds go to seed may reduce the contribution of these factors to IBK.

DISCLOSURE

The authors have no commercial or financial conflicts of interest or funding sources to declare.

REFERENCES

1. Vockeroth JR. Musca autumnalis De Geer in North America (Deptera: Muscidae). Can Entomol 1953;85:422–3.
2. Krafsur ES, Moon RD. Bionomics of the face fly, Musca autumnalis. Annu Rev Entomol 1997;42:503–23.
3. Krafsur ES, Moon RD, Kim Y, et al. Dynamics of diapause recruitment in populations of the face fly, Musca autumnalis. Med Vet Entomol 1999;13(4):337–48.
4. Barnett HC. The incrimination of arthropods as vectors of disease. Proc 11th Int Cong Entomol 1960;2:341–5.
5. Miller TA, Treece RE. Some relationship of face fly feeding, ovarian development, and incidence on dairy cattle. J Econ Entomol 1968;61:251–7.

6. Pickens LG, Miller RW. Biology and control of the face fly, musca autumnalis (diptera: muscidae). J Med Entomol 1980;17(3):195–210.

7. Turner EC, Hair JA. Effect of diet on longevity and fecundity of laboratory-reared face flies. J Econ Entomol 1967;60(3):857–60.

8. Lorincz G, Papp L, Kozma J. Computer simulation of the role of the face fly, Musca autumnalis, in spreading and causing infectious bovine keratoconjunctivitis (IBK), based on field data. Parasit Hung 1989;22:75–85.

9. Shugart JI. The face fly, Musca autumnalis Degeer: ability to cause mechanical damage and transmit pinkeye pathogens. J Econ Entomol 1978;72:633–5.

10. Giangaspero A, Broce AB. Micromorphology of the prestomal teeth and feeding behaviour of Musca autumnalis, M.larvipara and M.osiris (Diptera: Muscidae). Med Vet Entomol 1993;7(4):398–400.

11. Broce AB, Elzinga RJ. Comparison of prestomal teeth in the face fly (Musca autumnalis) and the house fly (Musca domestica) (Diptera: Muscidae). J Med Entomol 1984;21(1):82–5.

12. Parrish GV, Gerhard RR. Daily face fly infestation patterns of pastured beef cattle. Tenn Farm Home Sci 1976;97:12–3.

13. Benson OL, Wingo CW. Investigations of the face fly in Missouri. J Econ Entomol 1962;56(3):251–8.

14. Berkebile DR, Hall RD, Webber JJ. Field association of female face flies with Moraxella bovis, an etiological agent of bovine pinkeye. J Econ Entomol 1981;74(4):475–7.

15. Gerhardt RR, Allen JW, Greene WH, et al. The role of face flies in an episode of infectious bovine keratoconjunctivitis. J Am Vet Med Assoc 1982;180(2):156–9.

16. Arends JJ, Barto PB, Wright RE. Transmission of Moraxella bovis in the laboratory by the face fly (Diptera: muscidae). J Econ Entomol 1982;75(5):816–21.

17. Arends JJ, Wright RE, Barto PB, et al. Transmission of Moraxella bovis from blood agar cultures to Hereford cattle by face flies (Diptera: Muscidae). J Econ Entomol 1984;77(2):394–8.

18. Glass HW Jr, Gerhardt RR, Greene WH. Survival of Moraxella bovis in the alimentary tract of the face fly. J Econ Entomol 1982;75(3):545–6.

19. Glass HW Jr, Gerhardt RR. Recovery of Moraxella bovis (Hauduroy) from the crops of face flies (Diptera: Muscidae) fed on the eyes of cattle with infectious bovine keratoconjunctivitis. J Econ Entomol 1983;76(3):532–4.

20. Glass HW Jr, Gerhardt RR. Transmission of Moraxella bovis by regurgitation from the crop of the face fly (Diptera: Muscidae). J Econ Entomol 1984;77(2):399–401.

21. Cheng TH. Frequency of pinkeye incidence in cattle in relation to face fly abundance. J Econ Entomol 1967;60(2):598–9.

22. Steelman CD, Gbur EE, Tolley G, et al. Variation in population density of the face fly, Musca autumnalis De Geer, among selected breeds of beef cattle. J Agric Entomol 1993;10(2):97–106.

23. Gerhardt RR, Parrish GV, Snyder RQ, et al. Incidence of pinkeye in relation to face fly control. University of Tennessee, Knoxville, Tennessee: Tennessee Farm and Home Science; 1976. p. 14–5.

24. Cox PJ, Liddell JS, Mattinson AD. Infectious bovine keratoconjunctivitis: isolation of Moraxella bovis from two groups of young beef cattle in fly control field trials during 1981. Vet Rec 1984;115(2):29–32.

25. Tarry DW. Cattle fly control using controlled-release insecticides. Vet Parasitol 1985;18(3):229–34.

26. Allan J, Van Winden S. Randomised control trial comparing cypermethrin-based preparations in the prevention of infectious bovine keratoconjunctivitis in cattle. Animals (Basel) 2020;10(2):184.

27. Andresen CE, Loy DD, Brick TA, et al. Effects of extended-release eprinomectin on productivity measures in cow-calf systems and subsequent feedlot performance and carcass characteristics of calves. Transl Anim Sci 2019;3(1):273–87.

28. de Leon AAP, Mitchell RD, Watson DW. Ectoparasites of Cattle. Vet Clin N Amfood A 2020;36(1):173–+.

29. Freeman JC, Ross DH, Scott JG. Insecticide resistance monitoring of house fly populations from the United States. Pestic Biochem Phys 2019;158:61–8.

30. Heath A, Levot GW. Parasiticide resistance in flies, lice and ticks in New Zealand and Australia: mechanisms, prevalence and prevention. N Z Vet J 2015;63(4): 199–210.

31. Garros C, Bouyer J, Takken W, et al. Control of vector-borne diseases in the livestock industry: new opportunities and challenges. Ecol Cont Vector-bor 2018;5: 575–80.

32. Durel L, Estrada-Pena A, Franc M, et al. Integrated fly management in European ruminant operations from the perspective of directive 2009/128/EC on sustainable use of pesticides. Parasitol Res 2015;114(2):379–89.

33. Gerry AC. VetPestX: Database of pesticides for control of insect pests of animals. 2020. Available at: https://www.veterinaryentomology.org/vetpestx. Accessed September 29, 2020.

34. Coleman RE, Gerhardt RR. Isolation of moraxella bovis from the crops of field-collected face flies. J Agric Entomol 1987;4(1):92–4.

35. Hughes DE, Pugh GW Jr, McDonald TJ. Ultraviolet radiation and Moraxella bovis in the etiology of bovine infectious keratoconjunctivitis. Am J Vet Res 1965; 26(115):1331–8.

36. Pugh GW Jr, Hughes DE. Experimental production of infectious bovine keratoconjunctivitis: comparison of serological and immunological responses using pili fractions of Moraxella bovis. Can J Comp Med 1976;40(1):60–6.

37. Pugh GW Jr, Hughes DE, Schulz VD, et al. Experimentally induced infectious bovine keratoconjunctivitis: resistance of vaccinated cattle to homologous and heterologous strains of Moraxella bovis. Am J Vet Res 1976;37(1):57–60.

38. Angelos JA. Infectious bovine keratoconjunctivitis (pinkeye). Vet Clin North Am Food Anim Pract 2015;31(1):61–79, v-vi.

39. Alexander D. Infectious bovine keratoconjunctivitis: a review of cases in clinical practice. Vet Clin North Am Food Anim Pract 2010;26(3):487–503.

40. Brown MH, Brightman AH, Fenwick BW, et al. Infectious bovine keratoconjunctivitis: a review. J Vet Intern Med 1998;12(4):259–66.

41. Rogers DG, Cheville NF, Pugh GW Jr. Pathogenesis of corneal lesions caused by Moraxella bovis in gnotobiotic calves. Vet Pathol 1987;24(4):287–95.

42. Cullen AP. Photokeratitis and other phototoxic effects on the cornea and conjunctiva. Int J Toxicol 2002;21(6):455–64.

43. Vogelweid CM, Miller RB, Berg JN, et al. Scanning electron microscopy of bovine corneas irradiated with sun lamps and challenge exposed with Moraxella bovis. Am J Vet Res 1986;47(2):378–84.

44. Cullen AP. Ultraviolet induced lysosome activity in corneal epithelium. Albrecht Von Graefes Arch Klin Exp Ophthalmol 1980;214(2):107–18.

45. Pfister RR. The normal surface of corneal epithelium: a scanning electron microscopic study. Invest Ophthalmol 1973;12(9):654–68.

46. Chandler RL, Bird RG, Smith MD, et al. Scanning electron microscope studies on preparations of bovine cornea exposed to Moraxella bovis. J Comp Pathol 1983; 93(1):1–8.

47. Chandler RL, Smith K, Turfrey BA. Exposure of bovine cornea to different strains of Moraxella bovis and to other bacterial species in vitro. J Comp Pathol 1985; 95(3):415–23.

48. Jackman SH, Rosenbusch RF. In vitro adherence of Moraxella bovis to intact corneal epithelium. Curr Eye Res 1984;3(9):1107–12.

49. Lepper AW, Barton IJ. Infectious bovine keratoconjunctivitis: seasonal variation in cultural, biochemical and immunoreactive properties of Moraxella bovis isolated from the eyes of cattle. Aust Vet J 1987;64(2):33–9.

50. Hudson CD, Higgins HM, Huxley JN. Ocular complications of barren brome exposure in a suckler herd. Vet Rec 2006;159(12):388–9.

51. Bond W, Davies G, Turner R. The biology and non-chemical control of barren brome (Anisantha sterilis (L.) Nevski. Organic Gardens, Coventry, UK: HDRA Organic Publications Coventry; 2005.

Component Causes of Infectious Bovine Keratoconjunctivitis

The Role of Genetic Factors in the Epidemiology of Infectious Bovine Keratoconjunctivitis

Annette M. O'Connor, BVSc, MVSc, DVSc, FANZCVS

KEYWORDS

- Infectious bovine keratoconjunctivitis • Genetics • Heritability

KEY POINTS

- Very few estimates of heritability and quantitative trait locus (QTL) analysis are available for infectious bovine keratoconjunctivitis (IBK).
- The reported heritability of IBK is low to moderate.
- QTL on chromosome 1, 2, 12, 13, 20, and 21 have been associated with IBK resistance.

INTRODUCTION

When one thinks about the causes of disease, 1 approach to thinking of component causes is the epidemiologic triad: the pathogen or pathogens, the environment, and the host. Other articles in this special issue have evaluated component causes of the epidemiologic triad: the pathogen and the environment. With this article, the author evaluates the host with a particular focus on the genetic association with infectious bovine keratoconjunctivitis (IBK). In agriculture, breeding stock, plants, or animals that are resistant to a disease is one approach to control. The advantage of genetically resistant animals is that the effect is permanent, whereas other disease-prevention strategies might need to be continually reapplied. However, it is important when evaluating host genetics, as an approach to control that negative traits are not inadvertently introduced with the positive trait being developed.

One of the most interesting concepts from the host's perspective is the heritability of susceptibility or resistance to IBK. In reality, this is a challenging study question. Such studies require a large number of animals with known pedigree information.

Department of Large Animal Clinical Sciences, College of Veterinary Medicine, Michigan State University, 784 Wilson Road, Room G-100, East Lansing, MI 48824, USA
E-mail address: oconn445@msu.edu

Vet Clin Food Anim 37 (2021) 321–327
https://doi.org/10.1016/j.cvfa.2021.03.007
0749-0720/21/© 2021 Elsevier Inc. All rights reserved.

Fortunately, such populations do exist. One complicated part of the question is the measurement of the phenotype. Ideally, such studies would measure susceptibility or resistance to IBK. Instead, the phenotype that is studied is often detection of IBK or treatment of IBK. However, it is unclear how closely these measurable phenotypes represent the true genotype of interest, which is resistance or susceptible to IBK.

Furthermore, the fact that diagnosis of IBK or treatment of IBK can differ across studies also makes a comparison of estimates difficult. The metric commonly used to measure is heritability (h^2), which captures the proportion of phenotypic variation owing to genetic values that may include effects owing to dominance and epistasis. Heritability is formally defined as the proportion of phenotypic variation that is due to variation in genetic values.[1] Having determined if there is an element of heritability, the next step is to identify the loci correlated with the phenotypic trait and genes' function on the loci. For this article, a search was conducted to identify studies that have been undertaken to look at the host genetics of IBK. A citation search was conducted of [TS = ("infectious bovine keratoconjunctivitis" OR IBK OR pinkeye)] AND [DE = (cattle OR cattle diseases)] AND [TS = (genetic OR genome OR genomics OR inherit* OR heredit* OR gene)]. This search identified 39 citations, and these were screened for relevance to the topic. Nine studies[2–10] were found to be relevant. One additional study[11] was found because it was referenced by one of the nine.

HERITABILITY ESTIMATES

Fig. 1 plots the heritability point estimates and standard error (SE) from 4 studies. In this forest plot, each row represents a different point estimate of h^2. The central figure is a forest plot of the h^2 and the 95% confidence intervals. In each row, the black square represents the point estimate of h^2. Usually, for forest plots, the box's size represents the weight given to the observation in the pooled estimate; however, all the

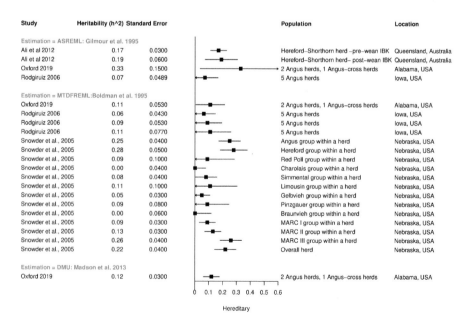

Study	Heritability (h^2)	Standard Error		Population	Location
Estimation = ASREML: Gilmour et al. 1995					
Ali et al 2012	0.17	0.0300		Hereford–Shorthorn herd –pre–wean IBK	Queensland, Australia
Ali et al 2012	0.19	0.0600		Hereford–Shorthorn herd– post–wean IBK	Queensland, Australia
Oxford 2019	0.33	0.1500		2 Angus herds, 1 Angus–cross herds	Alabama, USA
Rodgiruiz 2006	0.07	0.0489		5 Angus herds	Iowa, USA
Estimation = MTDFREML:Boldman et al. 1995					
Oxford 2019	0.11	0.0530		2 Angus herds, 1 Angus–cross herds	Alabama, USA
Rodgiruiz 2006	0.06	0.0430		5 Angus herds	Iowa, USA
Rodgiruiz 2006	0.09	0.0530		5 Angus herds	Iowa, USA
Rodgiruiz 2006	0.11	0.0770		5 Angus herds	Iowa, USA
Snowder et al., 2005	0.25	0.0400		Angus group within a herd	Nebraska, USA
Snowder et al., 2005	0.28	0.0500		Hereford group within a herd	Nebraska, USA
Snowder et al., 2005	0.09	0.1000		Red Poll group within a herd	Nebraska, USA
Snowder et al., 2005	0.00	0.0400		Charolais group within a herd	Nebraska, USA
Snowder et al., 2005	0.08	0.0400		Simmental group within a herd	Nebraska, USA
Snowder et al., 2005	0.11	0.1000		Limousin group within a herd	Nebraska, USA
Snowder et al., 2005	0.05	0.0300		Gelbvieh group within a herd	Nebraska, USA
Snowder et al., 2005	0.09	0.0800		Pinzgauer group within a herd	Nebraska, USA
Snowder et al., 2005	0.00	0.0600		Braunvieh group within a herd	Nebraska, USA
Snowder et al., 2005	0.09	0.0300		MARC I group within a herd	Nebraska, USA
Snowder et al., 2005	0.13	0.0300		MARC II group within a herd	Nebraska, USA
Snowder et al., 2005	0.26	0.0400		MARC III group within a herd	Nebraska, USA
Snowder et al., 2005	0.22	0.0400		Overall herd	Nebraska, USA
Estimation = DMU: Madson et al. 2013					
Oxford 2019	0.12	0.0300		2 Angus herds, 1 Angus–cross herds	Alabama, USA

0   0.1 0.2 0.3 0.4 0.5 0.6

Hereditary

Fig. 1. Estimates of heritability of IBK from published reports of pure and composite cattle breeds.[2,8,10,11]

boxes are the same size in this plot because the plot is descriptive. No pooled estimate was calculated, so no weighting was used. The horizontal lines through each black box represent the 95% confidence interval. These 95% confidence intervals were calculated using the *metagen* function in the meta package in R, based on the SE reported by the investigators.[12] Such an approach can mean the lower bound of the 95% confidence interval is negative; however, heritability cannot be less than zero. Therefore, **Fig. 1** truncates the lower bound of the 95% confidence interval at zero. The h^2 estimates might differ by population, model, or estimation method. The demographic information is reported in the columns of data on either side of the forest plot. The method of analysis is used as a subgroup, with analysis approaches grouped together.

The most extensive study that has been reported was conducted at the Meat Animal Research Center (MARC) in Nebraska, United States. The study reported on 20 years of data from more than 40,000 cattle. For 9 pure breeds, 3 composite breeds, and a pooled overall estimate, the investigators reported heritability estimates for IBK were very low, sometimes zero. The heritability estimates for Herefords (h^2: 0.28, SE: 0.05), Angus (h^2: 0.25, SE: 0.04) and a composite group created by the MARC known as MARC II (h^2: 0.26, SE: 0.04) were larger. These estimates are still low to moderate size. This study from the MARC is the only report publicly available that provided an insight into crossbreed comparisons in the same environment.

Other studies on a single breed in a single environment have been conducted. In 5 herds with Angus cattle in Iowa, the point estimates of heritability in those herd were around 0.1.[11] Rodriguez[11] looked at 2 statistical approaches and software packages to estimate heritability and found reasonably similar estimates across the multiple approaches. Using the same model with additive genetic and phenotypic efforts, the estimates from the ASREML approach[13] (h^2: 0.07, SE: 0.05) were very similar to those given by the MTDFREM approach (h^2: 0.11, SE: 0.08).[14] These analysis approaches are reported in **Fig. 1** by the subgroups, which indicate the statistical approach and the software package used for analysis reported by the investigators.[13–17] Rodriguez[11] also compared the impact of including different variance components with the MTDFREM approach, and there was little meaningful difference in the h^2 estimates as shown in **Table 1**.

Oxford[10] evaluated the heritability of IBK in calves from 2 purebred Angus and 1 Angus-derived herd in Alabama, United States. The data came from 3 continuous years, but the years appear not to be reported. Oxford[10] reported a moderate estimate of heritability (h^2: 0.33, SE: 0.15) based on the ASREML estimation method,[13] but lower estimates were obtained from DMU (h^2: 0.12, SE: 0.03)[17] and MTDFREM (h^2: 0.11, SE: 0.05).[14] However, the ASREML heritability estimate did have a great deal of uncertainty, as shown by the SE size (SE = 15).

Ali and colleagues[8] reported in 2013 a study that looked at a Hereford Shorthorn herd that has been developed for many years in tropical Queensland, Australia. The heritability estimates in this herd were h^2 = 0.19 when the outcome was IBK that occurred preweaning and h^2 = 0.17 when the outcome of interest was IBK occurring postweaning.

Kizilkaya and colleagues[9] report estimates of heritability of IBK for 3 different approaches to categorizing the disease. The study population was based on records of IBK collected from 860 animals born and raised in the Iowa State University Angus research herd from spring 2004 through spring 2008. Each animal's IBK status was determined at weaning time and was scored subjectively into 5 categories for left and right eyes. These data points were combined variously for 3 different metrics of IBK, as follows:

Table 1
Characteristics of studies reporting heritability estimates for infectious bovine keratoconjunctivitis

Author	Population	Random Effects/Variance Components in Models
Ali et al,[8] 2012	1 Hereford-Shorthorn herd in Queensland, Australia	Genetic
Oxford,[10] 2019	2 Angus herds and 1 Angus-derived herd in Alabama, United States	Additive genetic, environmental, and phenotypic
Rodriguez,[11] 2006	5 Angus herds in Iowa, United States	Additive genetic, phenotypic \ additive genetic, phenotypic, permanent environmental, maternal \ additive genetic, phenotypic, maternal
Snowder et al,[2] 2005	1 herd in Nebraska, United States with Angus, Hereford, Red Poll, Charolais, Simmental, Limousin, Gelbvieh, Pinzgauer, Braunvieh, MARC I, MARC II, MARC III	Additive genetic, phenotypic, maternal genetic, maternal permanent environmental

- Two categories ($c = 2$): 1 for both eyes unaffected and 2 otherwise.
- Three categories ($c = 3$): 1 for both eyes unaffected, 2 for a single affected eye, and 3 for both affected eyes.
- Nine categories ($c = 9$): Incidence was scored from 1 to 9 by adding the scores of the left and right eyes.

The approach to the analysis used by Kizilkaya and colleagues[9] differed from other studies because it used a BayesB threshold model.[18] Such an approach provides a posterior distribution of heritability, and so the results are not comparable to the frequentist approaches used by other investigators. However, the mean of the posterior distribution of the heritability reported in **Fig. 1** by Kizilkaya and colleagues[9] was similar to other estimates (0.064, 0.066, 0.0664) for the 2, 3, and 9 category models. The 2.5% and 97.5% posterior distribution intervals were (0.028, 0.116), (0.030, 0.115), and (0.029, 0.111) for the 2, 3, and 9 category models, respectively.

In summary, the overall picture from these studies is that Hereford and Angus cattle and their derivatives may have slightly higher heritability of IBK compared with other breeds. However, all of the investigators of the studies suggested that these heritability estimates were low or moderate and that using genetic selection approaches to modify the host to improve resistance to IBK would be slow. Furthermore, there are even fewer studies that evaluate any other adverse effects of resistance to IBK. For example, is there evidence in more than 1 study that resistance to IBK is positively or negatively correlated with other traits, such as average daily gain or feed conversion efficiency? Such data do not appear to be available other than the study conducted by Ali and colleagues[8] in Australia. However, this is just a single study, and therefore, it is difficult to extrapolate those results to the cattle population in general without any replication.

LOCI ASSOCIATED WITH INFECTIOUS BOVINE KERATOCONJUNCTIVITIS

Kizilkaya and colleagues[9] reported a study to detect single-nucleotide polymorphism (SNP) markers in linkage disequilibrium with genetic variants associated with IBK in

Angus cattle. High-density (53,367) SNP genotypes of purebred American Angus cattle were obtained using the Bovine SNP50 Infinium II BeadChip (Illumina, Inc, San Diego, CA, USA). Many SNPs were found for all 3 models, and these are reported in the original article. However, of interest is that 3 SNP windows ([109.01 Mb]–[109.87 Mb], [110.04 Mb]–[110.98 Mb], and [112.04 Mb]–[113.00 Mb]) on chromosome 1 overlapped the previously described quantitative trait locus (QTL) region for IBK susceptibility by others.[3] Interestingly, Kizilkaya and colleagues[9] reported that five 1-Mb SNP windows were identified as associated with IBK incidence (rs109448194–rs42270183 and rs41642303–rs110857971 on chromosome 2, rs108956311–rs43705367 on chromosome 12, rs29021773–rs109429649 on chromosome 13, and rs41966737–rs41640647 on chromosome 21). These SNP windows were found for all 3 models regardless of the IBK classification approach. Kizilkaya and colleagues[9] speculated that because these were found for all 3 models, there could be separate sets of genes controlling the occurrence and severity of IBK. Numerous candidate genes are reported in these windows, and a detailed discussion is available elsewhere.[9]

Casas and Stone[3] had previously reported the presence of QTL for IBK tolerance on chromosomes 1 and 20. Casas and Stone[4] further indicated that the region on chromosome 20 might be associated with a general resistance to bacterial diseases (including IBK) in a population of offspring from F1 sires: Brahman * Hereford (n = 547), Piedmontese * Angus (n = 209), Brahman * Angus (n = 176), and Belgian Blue * MARC III (n = 246). Interestingly, Kizilkaya and colleagues[9] did not find important factors on chromosome 20 for IBK incidence. Kizilkaya and colleagues[9] indicated that the difference in this result might be because of the difference in the *Bos taurus Bos indicus* nature of the population's studies. Kizilkaya and colleagues[9] studied a single herd with *B taurus* genetics, whereas Casas and Stone[3] and Casas and Snowder[4] studied a population with *B indicus * B taurus* genetics.

In a more recently published study about the association between chromosome 20 and IBK by the same group,[5] 539 F1 crossbred steers of *B taurus* decent (Angus, Hereford, Gelbvieh, Simmental, Charolais, Limousin, and Red Angus) were used to assess the association of SNP on BTA20 with IBK. The population was born in 1999 and 2000, with steers harvested in 2000 and 2001. Again, 5 regions were associated with IBK. The authors reported, *"Animals inheriting the minor allele genotype or the heterozygous genotype for marker BFGL-NGS-107368 were similar in their levels of IBK incidence, but had a significantly (P < 0.05) higher incidence of IBK than animals that inherited the major allele genotype. Animals that were homozygous for the minor allele genotype for markers BTA-51496-no-rs and BTB-01950117 had significantly different (P < .05) levels of IBK incidence than animals that inherited either the heterozygous genotype or the homozygous major allele genotype who were similar in their levels of IBK incidence. Furthermore, animals inheriting the homozygous minor allele genotypes from markers BFGL-NGA-92754 and rs17870710 were not significantly different in their levels of IBK incidence from animals inheriting the heterozygous or major allele genotypes. However, animals inheriting the heterozygous genotypes from these 2 markers had significantly lower rates of infection with IBK than animals inheriting the major allele genotype."*[5]

SUMMARY

In conclusion, as with the other aspects of the epidemiology of IBK, only a few studies have been conducted. However, the findings of the studies have generally been consistent. The h^2 of IBK resistance or susceptibility appears to be in the low range. Therefore, there may be candidates' genes associated with IBK occurrence and severity, but progress in controlling IBK with genetic approaches is likely to be slow.

DISCLOSURE

The author has nothing to disclose.

REFERENCES

1. Wray N, Visscher P. Estimating trait heritability. Nat Education 2008;1(1).
2. Snowder GD, Van Vleck LD, Cundiff LV, et al. Genetic and environmental factors associated with incidence of infectious bovine keratoconjunctivitis in preweaned beef calves. J Anim Sci 2005;83(3):507–18.
3. Casas E, Stone RT. Putative quantitative trait loci associated with the probability of contracting infectious bovine keratoconjunctivitis. J Anim Sci 2006;84(12): 3180–4.
4. Casas E, Snowder GD. A putative quantitative trait locus on chromosome 20 associated with bovine pathogenic disease incidence. J Anim Sci 2008;86(10): 2455–60.
5. Garcia MD, Matukumalli L, Wheeler TL, et al. Markers on bovine chromosome 20 associated with carcass quality and composition traits and incidence of contracting infectious bovine keratoconjunctivitis. Anim Biotechnol 2010;21(3): 188–202.
6. Kataria RS, Tait RG Jr, Kumar D, et al. Association of toll-like receptor four single nucleotide polymorphisms with incidence of infectious bovine keratoconjunctivitis (IBK) in cattle. Immunogenetics 2011;63(2):115–9.
7. Kizilkaya K, Tait RG, Garrick DJ, et al. Whole genome analysis of infectious bovine keratoconjunctivitis in Angus cattle using Bayesian threshold models. BMC Proc 2011;5(Suppl 4):S22.
8. Ali AA, O'Neill CJ, Thomson PC, et al. Genetic parameters of infectious bovine keratoconjunctivitis and its relationship with weight and parasite infestations in Australian tropical Bos taurus cattle. Genet Sel Evol 2012;44:22.
9. Kizilkaya K, Tait RG, Garrick DJ, et al. Genome-wide association study of infectious bovine keratoconjunctivitis in Angus cattle. BMC Genet 2013;14:23.
10. Oxford E. Estimation of genetic components related to infectious bovine keratoconjunctivitis susceptibility in Angus and Angus derived cattle produced in the Southern United States [Ph.D.]. Ann Arbor: University of Arkansas; 2019.
11. Rodriguez JE. Infectious bovine keratoconjunctivitis in Angus cattle [M.S.]. Ames, Iowa: Iowa State University; 2006.
12. Balduzzi S, Rucker G, Schwarzer G. How to perform a meta-analysis with R: a practical tutorial. Evid Based Ment Health 2019;22(4):153–60.
13. Gilmour A, Gogel B, Cullis B, et al. ASREML user guide release 3.0. Hemel Hempstead: VSN International Ltd; 2009.
14. Boldman KG, Kriese LA, Vleck LDV, et al. A manual for use of MTDFREML. A set of programs to obtain estimates of variances and covariances [DRAFT]. Washington, DC: U.S. Department of Agriculture, Agricultural Research Service; 1995.
15. Fischer TM, Gilmour AR, van der Werf JH. Computing approximate standard errors for genetic parameters derived from random regression models fitted by average information REML. Genet Sel Evol 2004;36(3):363–9.

16. Gilmour AR, Thompson R, Cullis BR. Average information REML: an efficient algorithm for variance parameter estimation in linear mixed models. Biometrics 1995;51(4):1440–50.
17. Madsen P, Jensen J. A user's guide to DMU—a package for analyzing multivariate mixed models. Version 6; release 5.2 2013. Available at: http://dmu. agrsci.dk.
18. Meuwissen THE, Hayes BJ, Goddard ME. Prediction of total genetic value using genome-wide dense marker maps. Genetics 2001;157(4):1819–29.

Evidence Base for Treatment of Infectious Bovine Keratoconjunctivitis

Annette M. O'Connor, BVSc, MVSc, DVSc, FANZCVS[a],*,
Mac Kneipp, BVSc, MVS, MANZCVS[b]

KEYWORDS

- Antibiotics • Infectious Bovine Keratoconjunctivitis
- Randomized control trials study design • Treatments

KEY POINTS

- Several antibiotics are available for treatment of infectious bovine keratoconjunctivitis (IBK) and evidence suggests these are effective.
- More research is needed to provide evidence for alternatives to antibiotics for treating IBK. No studies give information on the efficacy of these approaches, although they appear to be commonly used.
- The design of randomized controlled trial for treatments of IBK can be challenging.

BACKGROUND

Not all cattle with infectious bovine keratoconjunctivitis (IBK) are treated. The self-limiting tendency of the disease means the benefit of treating affected animals is questioned.[1] It has been estimated up to 50% of IBK cases in Australia are not treated[2]; however, IBK is painful,[3] and the possibility of severe outcomes increases without intervention, so treatment is recommended. Furthermore a systematic review and meta-analysis of the antibiotic treatment for IBK found treatment to be more effective than no treatment and results strongly indicated antibiotics of many kinds improved healing compared with placebo.[1] This is in keeping with ophthalmic principles, for conjunctivitis an antibacterial is appropriate, whereas treatment of IBK keratitis, an infected and therefore by definition a "complicated" corneal ulcer, involves treating the bacterial infection and any uveitis.[4]

Major considerations in treating IBK is whether medication will reach site of infection, have efficacy with a limited number of treatments, and is approved for use in

[a] Department of Large Animal Clinical Sciences, College of Veterinary Medicine, Michigan State University, 784 Wilson Road, Room G-100, East Lansing, MI 48824, USA; [b] Sydney School of Veterinary Science, The University of Sydney, Camden, NSW, Australia
* Corresponding author. Sydney School of Veterinary Science, The University of Sydney, Australia.
E-mail address: oconn445@msu.edu

Vet Clin Food Anim 37 (2021) 329–339
https://doi.org/10.1016/j.cvfa.2021.03.008
0749-0720/21/© 2021 Elsevier Inc. All rights reserved.
vetfood.theclinics.com

food-producing animals. Ophthalmic medications for IBK are delivered by topical, subconjunctival, or systemic routes, and each has advantages and disadvantages. The most used IBK treatments are antimicrobials; the eye ointment cloxacillin is particularly popular in Australia,[2] the subconjunctival (SJ) injection SJ penicillin may be the most commonly used treatment for IBK in the United States,[5] and parenteral antibiotics, like long-acting (LA) oxytetracycline (OTC).[6] Many other antibiotics have been used but few have been evaluated in controlled studies,[1,7,8] a particular issue because IBK may resolve without treatment.[1,9,10]

Nonantimicrobial treatments used against IBK include hypochlorous acid,[11] eye patches, and fly control. The latter was described as perhaps the most valuable treatment in outbreaks of IBK.[7] Ancillary IBK treatments are normally the domain of veterinarians and include atropine, corticosteroids, nonsteroidal anti-inflammatories, autologous serum, and surgery, such as tarsorrhaphy and eye ablation.

NORTH AMERICAN REGISTERED ANTIBIOTIC TREATMENTS FOR INFECTIOUS BOVINE KERATOCONJUNCTIVITIS
Oxytetracycline

In the United States, injectable oxytetracycline is registered for the treatment of IBK. A single dose of 9 mg oxytetracycline per pound of body weight administered intramuscularly or subcutaneously is the dose registered in the United States. The earliest Food and Drug Administration (FDA) freedom of information summary (NADA 113–232) does not provide supportive evidence of efficacy from randomized controlled trials for the treatment of IBK. In a review of all antibiotics assessed for IBK treatment, Cullen and colleagues[1] reported that a single study[12] was available that assesses injectable oxytetracycline at the label recommended dose compared with a placebo. The outcome the study used was the healing time, which was shorter for oxytetracycline; however, the effect size was not reported.

Tulathromycin

Tulathromycin is the only other product registered for the treatment of IBK in the United States, and the FDA Freedom of Drug summary provides strong evidence this product is effective. In 2 studies of naturally occurring IBK in male mixed breed beef calves, between 4 and 10 months of age, the evidence supports using tulathromycin. Calves were enrolled in the study when they had at least 1 clinical sign of IBK and the presence of an ulcer in 1 or both eyes. Eligible calves were grouped by corneal damage score, ranked by the number of clinical signs present, and then assigned to blocks of 2 animals each. The data from the 2 trials are presented in **Table 1**, and it can be seen that although the percentage recovery differs between the 2 studies, the comparative effect of tulathromycin is consistent.

Florfenicol

In Canada, florfenicol is registered for the treatment of IBK caused by *Moraxella bovis* at a dose of 40 mg/kg body weight (6 mL/45 kg) for subcutaneous injection; or by intramuscular injection at a dose of 20 mg/kg body weight (3 mL/45 kg), a total of 2 doses with a 48-hour interval should be given. The substantive evidence for product labeling does not seem to be publicly available in Canada; however, a peer-reviewed published study documented improved healing in florfenicol-treated animals: corneal ulcers healed by day 20 in 48 (98%) of 49 calves treated with florfenicol (20 mg/kg [9.1 mg/lb]) by intramuscular injection on day 0 and 2, 39 (93%) of 42 calves treated with florfenicol (40 mg/kg [18.2 mg/lb] of body weight) by subcutaneous injection, and 33 (63%) of 52 control calves.[13]

Table 1
Results of 2 studies in the substantive evidence for tulathromycin to Food and Drug Administration NADA 141-244

| Study Day | Number of Cures | |
	Tulathromycin: 2.5 mg/kg BW SC once	Saline: 0.025 mL/kg BW SC once
Study 1: Day 5	24/50	1/49
Study 1: Day 9	49/49	4/49
Study 1: Day 13	49/49	12/49
Study 1: Day 17	49/49	41/49
Study 1: Day 21	49/49	43/49
Study 2: Day 5	15/50	4/49
Study 2: Day 9	25/50	11/49
Study 2: Day 13	34/50	10/49
Study 2: Day 17	39/50	19/49
Study 2: Day 21	40/50	18/49

Abbreviation: BW SC, body weight subcutaneous.

Comparative Efficacy of Registered Antibiotic Treatments

One of the missing pieces of information about antibiotic treatments for IBK is the comparative efficacy. Ideally, veterinarians and producers would have such information to enable them to decide which of the antibiotics available to use. This information is not currently available from trials. The only study that directly compares 2 labeled antibiotic protocols comes from an outbreak of IBK in 30 Swiss Brown calves in Turkey.[14] The calves were randomly assigned into 2 equal groups (florfenicol or oxytetracycline). The animals received injections of florfenicol (20 mg/kg), intramuscular (IM), on hours 0 and 48, or injections of LA oxytetracycline (20 mg/kg), IM, on hours 0 and 48. The enrolled calves were kept indoors for 4 weeks and examined daily for the first week and then every 3 days for a further 3 weeks. Clinical recovery was assessed, and the remaining eye lesions were recorded at weekly intervals for 4 weeks. Treatment of the calves was considered to be successful when the ulcers completely healed within 4 weeks. The investigators reported that the mean (SEM) time of disappearance of corneal opacity was 13.14 (3.39) days in calves that received florfenicol and 18.56 (6.18) days in 9 of 15 calves that received oxytetracycline. Six calves treated with oxytetracycline still had small corneal lesions 4 weeks after treatment. It was not possible to reach a conclusion from the data provided, as the analyses likely needs to be a survival analysis with right-censored observations. Further, the study does not discuss the randomization approach, if the distribution of disease severity was even across the groups, or if the outcome assessment was blinded.

The report by Cullen and colleagues[1] included numerous other protocols for IBK; however, here, we focus on products labeled with registered antibiotic regimes in the United States or Canada.

OTHER TREATMENTS FOR INFECTIOUS BOVINE KERATOCONJUNCTIVITIS
Antibiotic Eye Ointments

The product Orbenin eye ointment is registered for use for IBK caused by *Mycobacterium bovis* in Australia. A search of the Centre for Agriculture and Bioscience International (CABI) abstract in Web of Science using the search string TS=("Orbenin" or benzathine cloxacillin") AND TS= ("infectious bovine keratoconjunctivitis" OR pinkeye) identified 2 published studies conducted in California. However, it is unknown if the formulation of the product tested in the United States in the 1990s is the same as the product registered in Australia.

Nonantibiotic Sprays

A search of the CABI abstract in Web of Science using the search sting TS=("Infectious bovine keratoconjunctivitis" OR pinkeye) AND TS=(patch OR patches) yielded 2 potentially relevant studies. Gard and colleagues[11] conducted a randomized, blinded controlled study which compared a commercially available 0.009% hypochlorous acid (Vetericyn PlusTM Pinkeye Spray) spray used topically onto each calf's cornea twice daily for 10 days compared with 2 mL of 0.9% saline also used topically onto each calf's cornea twice daily for 10 days. ImageJ software (NIH, Bethesda, MD) was used to determine the circumference, width, height, and area of all corneal lesions on a daily basis. The descriptive analysis provided percent change of the corneal lesion circumference and days to cure, visually suggesting that the hypochlorous acid treatment was associated with improved outcomes. However, the statistical analysis may have been conducted on different outcomes, that is, circumference, width, height, and area of the ulcers. The investigator did not report the effect sizes for these outcomes, only the results for the mean difference between groups: corneal lesion width (P = .0147), corneal lesion areas (P = .08), corneal lesion height (P = .11).

Another study reports assessing povidone-iodine spray.[15] The full text of the publication was not available. The results are unclear from the abstract because the effect sizes are not reported, nor are the results of hypothesis testing. The investigators reported, "*The severity of corneal lesions was assessed using a clinical scoring system and by measuring the surface areas of the corneal ulcers. The areas of the corneal lesions of all the calves in the three groups were significantly decreased. The mean corneal lesion areas for calves treated with povidone-iodine and oxytetracycline were significantly less than those in the controls at day 16. It is suggested that povidone-iodine spraying is an effective treatment for IBK in calves.*"

Eye Patches and Eyelid Flaps

Using an eye patch, eyelid flap, or other material to cover the eye is sometimes done to calves with IBK. However, it is unclear if the goal is to protect the eye from further irritation, decrease the spread of the organism, or promote faster healing. A search of the CABI in Web of Science using the search string TS=("Infectious bovine keratoconjunctivitis" OR pinkeye) AND TS=(patch OR patches OR eyelid OR eyelid) yielded no relevant studies. Therefore, there is no evidence available about the efficacy of eye patches or eyelid flaps for any of these possible purposes.

Bdellovibrio Bacteriovorus 109J

One novel treatment for IBK caused by *M bovis* is a biological, nonchemotherapeutic ophthalmic formulation that contains the predatory bacterium Bdellovibrio bacteriovorus 109J.[16] This treatment was assessed in a challenge study with 12 calves. The investigators concluded, "*Corneal ulcer size and severity and the time required for ulcer healing did not differ between the treatment and control groups.*"

DEVELOPING AN EVIDENCE BASE FOR TREATMENTS OF INFECTIOUS BOVINE KERATOCONJUNCTIVITIS

Effective prevention of IBK would be the ideal approach to the management of IBK. However, if effective prevention approaches are not available, then the next approach is to treat animals once the lesions have occurred. Evidence for effective treatment should come from the scientific process, which begins with a biologically sensible hypothesis and ends with multiple randomized, blinded controlled trials that measure the outcome of interest. Interestingly, as seen previously, the evidence base for treatments of IBK is quite small, even for the labeled products. Probably most important topics of interest include the following:

- Are there other treatment options that might be as effective as current options?
- Are there other treatment options that might be more suitable from one health perspective?
- What is the comparative efficacy of the products?

To answer these questions, thoughtfully designed and well-reported trials are needed.

CLINICAL EQUIPOISE

The first aspect of assessing treatment for IBK should be a reasonable and ethical hypothesis to test. In human health, there is debate[17–19] about the ethical framework for conducting a trial, and several approaches have been proposed, including clinical equipoise,[20–22] nonexploitation,[23] and net risk.[24] The debate is complicated and has not been reported from a veterinary perspective, but an essential component of the ethical frameworks is there must be a need for the study. Clinical equipoise is "*defined as a state of disagreement or uncertainty in the informed, expert medical community about the relative clinical merits of the intervention arms in a trial.*" In lay terms this is often interpreted as meaning "is it possible the null hypothesis is true?" Suppose it is known before the trial is conducted that the null hypothesis cannot be true. In that case, it is potentially unethical to allocate some study subjects to the inferior treatment knowingly. The question of who must think the null hypothesis could be true is often vaguely answered as "the medical community" rather than an individual. In veterinary science, discussions about ethical frameworks for conducting a trial are uncommon, perhaps because the evidence base is frequently small, and animal use complicates it. However, when embarking on a trial and selecting the comparisons of interest, researchers should consider the concept "Is it possible the null hypothesis is true?" Another aspect of this ethical framework is the need for the information. Suppose a large number of trials on a question have already been conducted. In that case, a meta-analysis might reveal that the effect of an intervention in known and additional trials will not contribute to the knowledge.

WHAT SHOULD THE REFERENT COMPARISON BE?

An aspect of the ethical framework for trials is the referent comparator.[25] We might expect an ethical framework for a trial to use the current standard of care as the referent comparison. This approach would use the baseline recovery risk as the comparison and minimize harms to participants. One rationale against always using the standard of care as the comparison group might be the absence of evidence that the standard care is superior to a nonactive placebo. The standard of care might have been adopted over time without proper evaluation.

Another factor when considering what referent comparator to use is the evidence network available. It will theoretically be possible to conduct the trial of interest and subsequently include it in a network meta-analysis.[26] Such an approach would allow indirect comparisons with other treatments in the network and potentially reduce the confidence interval around the effect size. If such an approach is envisioned, at least 2 treatments already included in the prior network should be included in the trial.

WHAT SHOULD BE THE EXPERIMENTAL COMPARATOR?

The experimental comparator(s) are usually predetermined and a much easier choice than determining the referent comparator. However, one often missed option is the idea of an additive treatment. For example, it might be of interest to know if adding a new treatment to an old treatment increases the efficacy. An example might be antibiotics compared with antibiotics with patches. Such a question asks if the addition of patches meaningfully adds to the efficacy of antibiotics. This study could be conducted as a pairwise comparison, or as a factorial design, with 4 groups: (1) antibiotics, (2) patches (3) antibiotic + patches, and (4) nonactive control (neither patches nor antibiotics). Much more information is gained from the factorial design, provided it is deemed ethical to have a nonactive control and the resources are available for a larger trial.

WHAT IS THE ALTERNATIVE HYPOTHESIS?

Having determined the referent comparator and the experimental comparator for the null hypothesis, the next question is the alternative hypothesis to be tested. Alternative hypotheses are generally considered to include options to test superiority, noninferiority, or equivalence, although that distinction can be debated.[27,28] In the traditional framework of alternative hypotheses, the choice is not without consequence. These options impact the sample size needed, and sample size impacts feasibility because larger trials are often not feasible.[28] Most clinical trials are conducted as superiority, as we are usually interested in knowing if the new treatment of interest is better than the current standard of care; however, superiority is traditionally conducted as a 2-sided test. Although the framework is that the new treatment is superior to the referent, the same sample size will test the new treatment being inferior for the same treatment difference.

ARTIFICIALLY INDUCED DISEASE OR NATURALLY OCCURRING DISEASE

Another choice to be made about assessing IBK treatments is whether to use naturally occurring disease or a challenge model. Certainly, most studies of antibiotic treatments use naturally occurring disease. This is likely because the sample sizes are larger. Although challenge models using UV light or scarification are well established, they are models of IBK rather than true IBK, so there are some external validity concerns.

APPROACH TO ALLOCATION TO TREATMENT

The study population for a treatment trial must be calves diagnosed IBK. For trial validity, it is essential that the treatment group are considered exchangeable, that is, the groups are evenly balance with respect to the distribution of measured and unmeasured confounders. Exchangeability is best achieved by simple randomization if the study is large enough. The qualifier is that often IBK trials are not large because the study population is only the herd population subset that develops IBK. With a small sample size, simple random allocation may not balance the most important confounder, disease severity, at enrollment.

It is often impractical in farm-based studies to look at calves daily, so disease duration might differ between calves at enrollment. For example, if the producers check the calves every 3 days, some calves may have day-old lesions and others 3-day-old lesions at enrollment. If only 30 calves are being allocated to the trial, an imbalance of disease severity across groups is feasible, and this imbalance could impact the outcome. A suggested approach is to block by disease severity and randomize within a block to control for this imbalance. Blocking by severity means that a randomization schedule is created for each severity level. Investigators use various severity scales. Although the severity scales may be imperfect, blocking by an imperfectly measured factor is preferable if the probability of disease severity unevenly balanced across groups is considered high. Block randomization adds more work for the person/people enrolling the calves, as it is necessary to assess the severity of the calves' IBK lesions before the treatment allocation can be unblinded, which is not needed for simple randomization. It would be critical that the person enrolling the calves is not aware of the next allocated treatment, as this could create a high risk of selection bias.

An alternative approach is to use a model of IBK in which the investigator induces disease on a known time frame. Because such studies are usually done in an experimental setting, observing calves frequently is more straightforward. After disease is induced, the researchers can set a trigger point determining when enrollment into the study occurs. For example, researchers might decide to start allocation to the treatments a specified time period after the disease is induced or at a set level of severity. One difficulty of such an approach is deciding the trigger point for enrollment and obtaining ethical approval for the trigger point. If the trigger point is too soon in the disease process, then the comparison between groups might be biased toward the null, and a meaningful outcome may be difficult to measure. Selecting a trigger point that is associated with severe lesions creates concerns about animal welfare.

WHAT OUTCOME TO ASSESS

What outcome to assess for a clinical trial is always important because it impacts the sample size needed and the validity. Outcomes that have been used include the following:.

- Cure (or no cure) at a certain number of days posttreatment.
- Weight gain at a certain number of days posttreatment.
- Clinical score at a certain number of days posttreatment
- The surface area of ulcers at a certain number of days posttreatment
- Number of days to cure

For all these outcomes except days to "cure," the "best" number of days posttreatment to compare the groups is unclear. Hence, repeated measurements are common in IBK. If the number of days is too soon, the treatment may not have had time to work. As most ulcers from IBK resolve without any treatment, any difference between treatments decreases as time increases. The data in **Table 1** illustrate the changing effect size by days.

Cure is a binary outcome; animals are categorized as either cured or not cured. The approach to reporting clinical cure should be the proportion of animals in each group and a comparative measure such as risk ratio or incidence odds ratio. An approach to reporting a binary outcome is provided in **Table 2**. The risk ratio for a cure is 1.23 with a 95% confidence interval of 1.03–1.46. This estimate shows that the risk of a cure is 1.23-fold higher in the group treated with A compared with the group treated with B. The confidence interval suggests some uncertainty because it is quite wide, but it is a consistently positive effect.

Table 2
Comparison of the effect size and confidence interval when perfect diagnosis compared with nondifferential imperfect sensitivity in the diagnosis of infectious bovine keratoconjunctivitis (IBK) and bias toward the null

Treatment	Cured	Not Cured	Risk Ratio
100% sensitivity, 100% specificity of IBK cure diagnosis			
Treatment A	80	20	
Treatment B	65	35	1.23 (1.03–1.46)
90% sensitivity, 100% specificity of IBK cure diagnosis			
Treatment A	72	28	
Treatment B	59	41	1.22 (0.99–1.49)

How investigators define a cure can vary greatly, and for IBK research, a standard metric of cure has not been established. Some investigators might define a cure as no fluorescein uptake; others might define it as an ulcer less than a particular size, or a scar, or no blepharospasm. Imperfect definition of a cure has 2 impacts. First, if there is differential diagnosis of the cure, which would occur if outcome assessment was not properly blinded, then the bias can be in any direction. However, the expectation is that the bias would be away from the null. If the measurement is imperfect but nondifferential, then the concern is a loss of power. As shown in **Table 2**, when the sensitivity is imperfect, the effect size is closer to the null effect, and the confidence interval increases in width. The bias toward the null would be even larger if specificity was also imperfect.

The surface area of the eye and weight gain are both continuous outcomes. The mean surface area, perhaps transformed to be normally distributed, or the mean weight gain (or final weight) should be reported for both groups. As the outcome is continuous, there is no set relationship between the standard error and the mean, therefore for these truly continuous outcomes, the standard error of the group mean should also be reported, as well as the number of animals in each group. The effect size should be reported as the mean difference and the standard error of the mean difference or the 95% confidence interval. If there is no difference in either treatment on the outcome, the mean difference will be close to zero.

Clinical score is an ordinal outcome that is, commonly used for IBK. Regrettably, for IBK trials, clinical score analyses often ignore the ordinal nature of clinical score data, a common concern in veterinary science.[29–31] Most studies treat clinical score data as continuous, making the assumption that the change in scales is linear, that is, assuming that the difference between a clinical score of 1 and 2 is the same as a clinical score of 3 and 4. Obviously, this cannot be known.

In **Table 3**, 3 hypothetical examples of clinical score data are presented. Notice that the mean score per group is the same when the numerical values are averaged. However, looking at the definition of the scores, it appears there are differences. For example, the comparison of the category frequency in scenario 1 compared with scenario 2 suggests more severe disease in scenario 2. Further, the difference is the ordinal scales between Scenarios 1 and 2 compared with scenario 3 is lost when the numerical averages are used. A tutorial on approaches to hypothesis testing for ordinal data is not the purpose of this article; however, if the decision is made to use ordinal data, several references on how these data should be analyzed are available.[29–31] These articles often focus on hypothesis testing rather than estimation of the effect and often propose nonparametric tests. However, investigators should consider how they present ordinal data. Investigators are encouraged to present the frequency of the categories, the definitions of the scores, rather than just the number, and use an

Table 3
Impact of clinical scores in hiding important differences in data within and between studies

Disease Severity	Numerical Value Attached	Number #Treatment A	Number #Treatment B	Treatment A	Treatment B	Risk Ratio Risk A/Risk B
Nothing	1	10	10	10	10	
Mild	2	10	15	20	30	0.83(0.48–1.43)
Moderate	3	10	5	30	15	1.5 (0.64–3.47)
Severe	4	10	10	40	40	1 (0.53–1.85)
Mean score				Mean =(100/40) = 2.5	Mean = (95/40) = 2.375	
Nothing	1	10	10	10	10	1 (0.53–1.85)
Mild	2	10	10	20	20	0.83 (0.48–1.43)
Moderate	3	10	15	30	45	1.5 (0.64–3.47)
Severe	4	10	5	40	20	
				Mean = (100/40) = 2.5	Mean = (95/40) = 2.375	
Nothing	1	10	10	10	10	0.83 (0.48–1.43)
Moderate	2	10	15	20	30	1.5 (0.64–3.47)
Severe	3	10	5	30	15	1 (0.53–1.8)
Blind	4	10	10	40	40	
				Mean = (100/40) = 2.5	Mean = (95/40) = 2.375	

effect size in an understandable metric for the end-user. In **Table 3**, the risk ratio is compared with the baseline, and such an approach is often interpretable to the reader. Similarly, graphic representation of ordinal data can help readers understand the data rather than nonparametric *P* values.

SUMMARY

In conclusion, there is a small amount of evidence that product-labeled antibiotic treatments are effective compared with no treatment. However, many questions remain about how the veterinary community should be treating IBK cases. Can we find approaches that reduce antibiotic use or reduce the type of antibiotic used? What is the comparative efficacy of the available options? Designing trials for the treatment of IBK is somewhat more challenging than designing trials to assess vaccines, mainly because of the potential for the confounding effect of disease severity at enrollment and the question of referent comparator. However, producers and veterinarians will immediately use new high-quality trials providing better information about commonly used treatment options such as patches, third-eyelid flaps, and so forth.

DISCLOSURE

Both the authors have nothing to disclose.

REFERENCES

1. Cullen JN, Yuan C, Totton S, et al. A systematic review and meta-analysis of the antibiotic treatment for infectious bovine keratoconjunctivitis: an update. Anim Health Res Rev 2016;17(1):60–75.
2. Kneipp M, Govendir M, Laurence M, et al. Current incidence, treatment costs and seasonality of pinkeye in Australian cattle estimated from sales of three popular medications. Prev Vet Med 2020;187:105232.
3. Dewell RD, Millman ST, Gould SA, et al. Evaluating approaches to measuring ocular pain in bovine calves with corneal scarification and infectious bovine keratoconjunctivitis–associated corneal ulcerations. J Anim Sci 2014;92:1161–72.
4. Maggs DJ. Diseases cornea and sclera. In: Maggs DJ, Miller PE, Ofri R, editors. Slatter's fundamentals of veterinary ophthalmology. 6th edition. St Louis (MO): Elsevier; 2018. p. 213–53.
5. Angelos JA. Infectious bovine keratoconjunctivitis (pinkeye). Vet Clin North Am Food Anim Pract 2015;31:61–79.
6. Smith JA, George LW. Treatment of acute ocular *Moraxella bovis* infections in calves with parenterally administered long-acting oxytetracyline formulation. Am J Vet Res 1985;46(4):840–7.
7. George LW. Clinical infectious Bovine Keraotconjunctivitis. Compend Contin Educ Dent 1984;6(12):712–22.
8. O'Connor AM, Wellman NG, Evans RB, et al. A review of randomized clinical trials reporting antibiotic treatment of infectious bovine keratoconjunctivitis in cattle. Anim Health Res Rev 2006;7(1/2):119–27.
9. Cox JE. Large-animal ophthalmology. Vet Rec 1969;84:526–33.
10. Alexander D. Infectious Bovine Keratoconjunctivitis: a review of cases in clinical practice. Vet Clin North Am 2010;26(3):487–503.
11. Gard J, Taylor D, Maloney R, et al. Preliminary evaluation of hypochlorous acid spray for treatment of experimentally induced infectious bovine keratoconjunctivitis. The Bovine Practitioner 2016;50(2):180–9.

12. George L, Mihalyi J, Edmondson A, et al. Topically applied furazolidone or parenterally administered oxytetracycline for the treatment of infectious bovine keratoconjunctivitis. J Am Vet Med Assoc 1988;192(10):1415–22.
13. Angelos JA, Dueger EL, George LW, et al. Efficacy of florfenicol for treatment of naturally occurring infectious bovine keratoconjunctivitis. J Am Vet Med Assoc 2000;216(1):62–4.
14. Gokce HI, Citil M, Genc O, et al. A comparison of the efficacy of florfenicol and oxytetracycline in the treatment of naturally occurring infectious bovine keratoconjunctivitis. Ir Vet J 2002;55(11):573–6.
15. Seifi HA, Rad M, Madadi MS. Povidone iodine spray for treatment of infectious bovine keratoconjunctivitis. Journal of the Faculty of Veterinary Medicine 2001; 56(1):Pe97–100. University of Tehran.
16. Boileau MJ, Mani R, Breshears MA, et al. Efficacy of Bdellovibrio bacteriovorus 109J for the treatment of dairy calves with experimentally induced infectious bovine keratoconjunctivitis. Am J Vet Res 2016;77(9):1017–28.
17. London AJ. Social value, clinical equipoise, and research in a public health emergency. Bioethics 2019;33(3):326–34.
18. Rabinstein AA, Brinjikji W, Kallmes DF. Equipoise in clinical trials: angst and progress. Circ Res 2016;119(7):798–800.
19. Is the concept of clinical equipoise still relevant to research? BMJ 2018;360: k1065.
20. Miller FG. Clinical equipoise and risk-benefit assessment. Clin Trials 2012;9(5): 621–7.
21. Miller FG. Equipoise and the ethics of clinical research revisited. Am J Bioeth 2006;6(4):59–61 [discussion: W42-55].
22. Freedman B. Equipoise and the ethics of clinical research. N Engl J Med 1987; 317(3):141–5.
23. Buchanan D, Miller FG. Principles of early stopping of randomized trials for efficacy: a critique of equipoise and an alternative nonexploitation ethical framework. Kennedy Inst Ethics J 2005;15(2):161–78.
24. Rid A, Wendler D. A framework for risk-benefit evaluations in biomedical research. Kennedy Inst Ethics J 2011;21(2):141–79.
25. Brower RG, Bernard G, Morris A, et al. Ethics and standard of care in clinical trials. Am J Respir Crit Care Med 2004;170(2):198–9 [author reply: 199].
26. Nikolakopoulou A, Mavridis D, Salanti G. Using conditional power of network meta-analysis (NMA) to inform the design of future clinical trials. Biom J 2014; 56(6):973–90.
27. Dunn DT, Copas AJ, Brocklehurst P. Superiority and non-inferiority: two sides of the same coin? Trials 2018;19(1):499.
28. Blackwelder WC. "Proving the null hypothesis" in clinical trials. Control Clin Trials 1982;3(4):345–53.
29. Boden L. Clinical studies utilising ordinal data: pitfalls in the analysis and interpretation of clinical grading systems. Equine Vet J 2011;43(4):383–7.
30. Osterstock JB, MacDonald JC, Boggess MM, et al. Technical note: analysis of ordinal outcomes from carcass data in beef cattle research. J Anim Sci 2010; 88(10):3384–9.
31. Plant JD, Giovanini JN, Villarroel A. Frequency of appropriate and inappropriate presentation and analysis methods of ordered categorical data in the veterinary dermatology literature from January 2003 to June 2006. Vet Dermatol 2007;18(4): 260–6.

The Evidence Base for Prevention of Infectious Bovine Keratoconjunctivitis Through Vaccination

Gabriele Maier, DVM, MPVM, PhD, DACVPM[a],
Annette M. O'Connor, BVSc, MVSc, DVSc, FANZCVS[b],*,
David Sheedy, DVM, MPVM[c]

KEYWORDS

- Infectious bovine keratoconjunctivitis • Vaccine • Prevention • *Moraxella bovis*
- *Moraxella bovoculi*

KEY POINTS

- Although the quality of publications for infectious bovine keratoconjunctivitis (IBK) vaccines has improved over time, no trials report effective commercially available vaccines.
- IBK is a multifactorial disease, which may explain the lack of successful prevention methods targeting a single cause.
- Antigenicity of *Moraxella* spp and immune responses are complex in nature, and some conflicting evidence exists surrounding the importance of individual components.

INTRODUCTION

Although treatment for infectious bovine keratoconjunctivitis (IBK) can be effective and rapidly resolve lesions, prevention of IBK is a major goal for producers and veterinarians alike. Currently, prevention of IBK has primarily focused on the search for an effective vaccine, with *Moraxella bovis* being the only targeted pathogen until the recent development of *Moraxella bovoculi* vaccines following its identification in 2007.[1] This article discusses in order: possible targets for vaccines, the immune response of the host, available evidence for the efficacy of vaccines followed by a discussion of the reasons for failure of experimental studies to translate to field trials, and finally, a discussion of criteria to assess the quality of vaccine trial studies for IBK.

[a] Department of Population Health & Reproduction, School of Veterinary Medicine, University of California Davis, Davis, 1 Shieds Avenue, VM3B, Davis, CA 95616, USA; [b] Department of Large Animal Clinical Sciences, College of Veterinary Medicine, Michigan State University, 784 Wilson Road Room D-204, East Lansing, MI 48824-1314, USA; [c] Veterinary Medicine Teaching and Research Center, School of Veterinary Medicine, University of California Davis, 18830 Road 112, Tulare, CA 93274, USA
* Corresponding author.
E-mail address: oconn445@msu.edu

Vet Clin Food Anim 37 (2021) 341–353
https://doi.org/10.1016/j.cvfa.2021.03.009
0749-0720/21/© 2021 Elsevier Inc. All rights reserved.

POSSIBLE VACCINE TARGETS FOR *MORAXELLA BOVIS*

Two proteins have been identified as necessary for pathogenicity of *M bovis*: pili and cytotoxins. Pili are necessary for adherence of the bacteria to corneal epithelium, whereas cytotoxins are responsible for degradation of corneal epithelium and lysis of leukocytes. Many *M bovis* vaccines have pili or cytotoxins as their antigenic target.

Pili or Fimbriae

Pili are filamentous structures expressed on the ends of some gram-negative bacteria that enable them to adhere to cell surfaces, which is a prerequisite for many bacterial diseases,[2] and are considered virulence factors.[3] *M bovis* pili have been categorized into 7 non-cross-reacting serogroups (A to G).[4] Furthermore, pili production can be differentiated based on colony morphology.[5,6] Two types of pilin polypeptide subunits, which make up pili, have been identified: The Q (Quick) pilin has been suggested to be specific for colonization of the cornea, whereas the I (Intermediate) pilin appears to help maintain an established infection.[7,8] Phenotypic expression of pilin is subject to phase variation, that is, the same bacteria seem capable of expressing more than 1 pilin type through a gene inversion event, which may enable them to evade a host immune response directed toward pili.[9,10]

There is ample empirical evidence for a contribution of pili in the pathogenicity of *M bovis* as well as for the role of pili as an extracellular antigen eliciting an immune response..[11–14] Calves experimentally infected with cultures of *M bovis* grown in the piliated phase developed higher lesion scores than those infected with the same culture of *M bovis* grown in the nonpiliated phase.[12,13] Immunization with a piliated *M bovis* bacterin resulted in fewer IBK cases after challenge with the piliated homologous strain compared with controls.[12,13]

However, *M bovis* pili vaccines have failed to provide cross-protection to heterologous pili serogroups,[14] and inclusion of multiple serogroups into a single vaccine is thought to result in antigenic competition where titers to each serogroup of pili are insufficient to result in immune protection.[15] Similarly, in footrot vaccines, which target pili of the causative agent *Dichelobacter nodosus*, multivalent vaccines resulted in 25% to 30% of serum antibody titers reached with a monovalent vaccine, and were associated with a linear decrease in protection.[16–18] In experimental challenge studies, there is evidence for protection from lesion development to different *M bovis* strains by pili vaccines though, as long as the strains belong to the same serogroup.[19] Within a bacterial species, strains are genetic variants, whereas serogroups share common antigens. Pili genes have been successfully cloned into *Pseudomonas aeruginosa*, and derived pili used in an experimental recombinant vaccine, which showed similar efficacy to a pili vaccine produced from *M bovis* cells of the same strain.[20]

Cytotoxins

Hemolytic strains of *M bovis* secrete an RTX (repeats in structural toxin) cytotoxin, also called cytolysin or hemolysin. The toxin lyses bovine neutrophils, erythrocytes, lymphocytes, and corneal epithelial cells, resulting in corneal ulceration.[21–23] Nonhemolytic strains and supernatants from nonhemolytic strains are avirulent.[21,24] Hemolysin antibodies capable of neutralizing hemolysin from diverse *M bovis* strains develop in cattle with IBK.[25–28] The sequence of the cytotoxin gene (*mbxA*) is highly conserved between geographically diverse *M bovis* isolates within the United States[29] and is an attractive target for *M bovis* vaccines.

The first experimental vaccine specifically targeting the hemolysin cytotoxin using cell-free supernatant was tested in 1994.[27] The small, nonrandomized, nonblinded study found lower cumulative incidence of IBK after exposure to a heterologous challenge strain in calves vaccinated with a hemolytic strain than a nonhemolytic strain or nonvaccinated controls, but no difference from a recombinant pili vaccine.

Field studies with experimental (not commercial) cytotoxin vaccines have used either culture supernatant or recombinant vaccines and have yielded mixed results where the vaccinates had a lower cumulative incidence of IBK[30] than controls or where no difference was detected between groups.[25,31] At present, no vaccines directed at cytotoxins only are commercially available.

LOCAL VERSUS SYSTEMIC IMMUNE RESPONSES

A vaccine is expected to elicit an immune response that protects the animal from infection. Despite numerous studies, there is no consensus or clear evidence as to the importance of local versus systemic immunity to M bovis or which immunoglobulins confer protective ocular immunity. The discussion on the importance of local versus systemic immunity to IBK stems from the fact that the cornea is not vascularized, and this limits humoral antibodies' access to the cornea.[32] Bovine corneal defenses to bacterial infections include the precorneal tear film, lactoferrin,[33] a local antibody response through secretory immunoglobulin A (sIgA), and a systemic antibody response through the selective transfer of IgG1 from serum to tears.[14,25,34] However, the evidence for the importance of lacrimal antibodies in IBK immunity is conflicting; although sIgA and IgG become elevated in calves with IBK,[25,35] they may not protect against developing clinical IBK.[36–39] One reason for disagreements on the role of local immune responses in IBK may be that most studies did not control for total immunoglobulin isotype levels in samples, which may fluctuate between individuals. Controlling for total antibody isotype levels in serum or tears would make antigen-specific antibody isotype levels more meaningful.[25] If the metric for local immune response versus systemic was standardized to account for individual differences in absolute levels, that is, controlling for total immunologic levels, the results of studies on this topic might be easier to understand and compare. If local immunity is found to be important for a protective response, it would support developing mucosal routes of vaccine administration (eg, intranasal, subconjunctival, aerosolized to the eye surface) that elicit a strong local immune response.

Attempts to discern whether subconjunctival injection leads to improved immunity over parenteral injection led to mixed results.[40–42] Direct comparison between subconjunctival vaccine studies is difficult because of different outcomes being measured between these studies. Given the difficulty of administering subconjunctival injections and the potential for conjunctival and blepharal swelling postinoculation, this avenue of research has the potential to be limited by the ability to commercialize a vaccine that requires a subconjunctival injection.

The evidence for the suitability of aerosolized ocular or intranasal vaccines is sparse. The 2 experimental studies published in 1994 on aerosolized fimbrial vaccines showed the aerosolized delivery to be as efficacious as the subcutaneous delivery in preventing clinical IBK.[43,44] Experimental intranasal vaccines elicit a lacrimal sIgA response but have not yet produced evidence for vaccine efficacy.[45,46] At present, no commercial vaccines are labeled for aerosolized or intranasal use, and no published field trials for aerosolized or intranasal IBK vaccines exist.

An argument proposed against the use of systemic vaccines is that IgG, the predominant isotype stimulated by systemic vaccination, could result in complement fixation and attract neutrophils into the corneal stroma leading to more severe lesions, as was observed in 1 study.[25]

PREVENTION OF *MORAXELLA BOVIS* INFECTION OF THE CORNEA OR ELIMINATION OF THE CARRIER STATUS

M bovis appears to be as abundant in the ocular microbiome of calves that develop IBK as it is in calves that do not.[47] Based on the limited available evidence, asymptomatic carriers do not have detectable serum[48] or lacrimal[35] antibodies to *M bovis* antigen, and elimination of the carrier status by vaccination or use of antimicrobials does not appear feasible. Hughes and Pugh[49] did not find evidence that their vaccines prevented the establishment of *M bovis* in the eye of experimentally challenged cattle.[50] One-time treatment of pregnant females with tilmicosin, a macrolide antibiotic, to eliminate carrier status before parturition with the intent of protecting offspring from IBK did not decrease incidence of IBK in calves[51] and does not comply with today's recommendations for judicious use of antimicrobials.

THE ROLE OF MATERNAL ANTIBODIES AND TRANSFER OF PASSIVE IMMUNITY

Age has consistently been found to be a risk factor for IBK, for example, in a single herd observed over 5 years, younger calves were more susceptible to develop IBK than older ones, and has been mainly attributed to a lack of active immunity in the younger calves.[52–56] There is also limited evidence that younger calves are more likely to develop severe signs of IBK, and duration of infection is increased.[57] Evidence exists in support of effective passive immunity[44,50,58] and against it.[51]

EFFICACY OF COMMERCIALLY AVAILABLE VACCINES FOR INFECTIOUS BOVINE KERATOCONJUNCTIVITIS

In the United States, there are 3 types of vaccines commercially available to prevent IBK: licensed vaccines, conditionally licensed vaccines, and autogenous vaccines. The only publicly available randomized controlled trials that clearly assessed commercially available licensed vaccines targeted at *M bovis* were conducted in the late 1980s[59] and 2015.[60] The late 1980s study reported no statistically significant difference in the incidence of clinical IBK; however, the effect size was not reported. The 2015 study reported no protective effect of the vaccine: IBK was detected in 65 from 110 (59.1%) vaccinated calves and 62 from 104 (59.6%) unvaccinated calves (unadjusted risk ratio, 0.99; 95% confidence interval, 0.79–1.24) during the study period (**Fig. 1**). No significant difference in weaning weights was identified between vaccinated and unvaccinated calves (unadjusted effect size, 4.40 kg [9.68 lb]; 95% confidence interval, −3.46 to 12.25 kg [−7.61–26.95 lb]).

A study on a conditionally licensed *M bovoculi* vaccine became available in 2019.[61] The results of that 2-year (2017–2018) study suggested the vaccine was not protective and may increase risk of IBK. In both years of the study, calves receiving the vaccine had more IBK. This effect was small. The pooled risk ratio was 1.30 (95% confidence interval, 0.84–2.01). The pooled unadjusted difference in mean weight (kg) at weaning was −0.88 (95% confidence interval, −7.2–5.43) (see **Fig. 1**).

Autogenous vaccines are manufactured from bacterial strains isolated from diseased animals for use in the herd where the diseased animal originated. They are intended for use when no commercially licensed product is available or when commercially licensed products have not provided adequate protection. Autogenous vaccines are manufactured at licensed facilities under United States Department of Agriculture oversight, and several companies offer the service for the manufacture of pinkeye vaccines, which are popular with practitioners and producers. However, scientific evidence as to the efficacy of autogenous vaccines for different agents

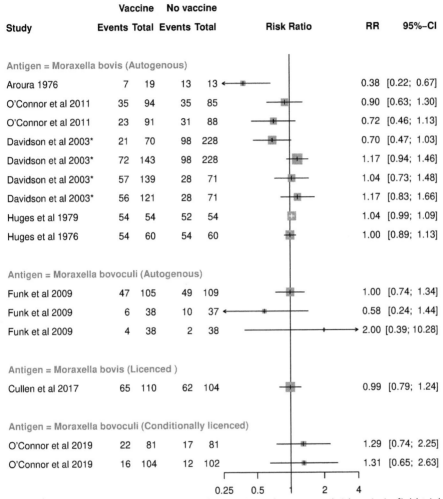

Fig. 1. Frequency of IBK in vaccinated and unvaccinated groups and risk ratio in field trials of commercially available vaccines. For the risk ratio (RR), the vaccinated data are in the numerator, so an RR less than 1 indicated a protective effect for vaccination, greater than 1 indicated the control is protective. [a] A pairwise comparison from a 3-arm trial, that is, controls repeated. CI, confidence interval.[79]

implicated in causing IBK is completely lacking to date. A meta-analysis of available vaccine trials with autogenous *M bovis* vaccines for the prevention of IBK found 9 pairwise comparisons in 4 published studies, none of which found a significant association between vaccination with an autogenous *M bovis* vaccine and the risk of developing IBK[42,62–65] (see **Fig. 1**).

EFFICACY OF EXPERIMENTAL VACCINATION

Overwhelmingly, experimental studies of *M bovis* vaccine candidates have documented that experimental vaccines are able to reduce the outcome of interest in challenge studies or field trials.[66] An older review found that most of the assessed noncommercial candidates reported an effect size less than 1, which was indicative of a protective effect.[66] There is also a limited number of studies for vaccines that target non-*M bovis* pathogens, including *Mycoplasma bovoculi* or *M bovoculi*. None have reported a protective effect of a vaccine against clinical disease. A whole-cell extract or inactivated whole-cell vaccine for *M bovoculi* did not offer any advantage compared with unvaccinated calves, as all calves cleared the organism after challenge with 10^8 units of *M bovoculi* suspension 3 weeks following vaccination.[58] Although *M bovoculi* has not been shown to meet the characteristics of a causal organism, it is commonly isolated from IBK-associated corneal ulcers, where *M bovis* was unable to be cultured.[1,67,68] There are currently no published *M bovoculi* vaccine studies that show a reduction in IBK incidence. Field vaccination with an experimental recombinant ISCOM matrix adjuvanted *M bovoculi* cytotoxin subunit vaccine did not achieve differences in the cumulative proportion of corneal ulcers between vaccinates and adjuvant-injected controls.[69] An experimental vaccine combining antigens from both *M bovis* and *M bovoculi* was also not able to show differences between IBK incidence of vaccinated and control calves.[31]

FAILURE OF RESULTS FROM EXPERIMENTAL VACCINES TO TRANSLATE TO COMMERCIAL PRODUCTS

Although initial experimental challenge studies for many vaccine candidates have shown promising results for the efficacy of various vaccines, few have been assessed in field trials or the promising results could not be replicated in field studies.[70] There are many reasons for the failure of translation, clinical and methodological. Possible clinical explanations for field trial vaccine efficacy failure include the following:

- The presence of antigenically different pathogen strains from the vaccine strain in naturally occurring disease.[69,70]
- The presence of another causal organisms.[33] This argument would hold only if the target organism for the vaccine was absent or had little influence, because one would still expect a lessening effect if the target organism's contribution was reduced by a vaccine.
- Insufficient time between vaccination and exposure to *M bovis*. The magnitude and duration of the immune response for each vaccine will depend on factors such as vaccine antigen, adjuvant,[71] number of inoculations, or route of administration.[72] A balance must be struck between providing enough time for the body to develop an immune response and the waning of titers with time, while fitting vaccinations into the production schedule and aligning with the summer pinkeye season. Vaccine field trials that miss the best window of opportunity may suffer from low efficacy, but one might also question the practicality of a vaccine if the timing of vaccinations must line up with these timepoints precisely.
- A vaccine strain that is not very antigenic.[69,70,73]
- Increased herd immunity conferred to nonvaccinates by vaccinates, that is, less frequent transmission or survival rate of *Moraxella* organisms in eyes of calves in the vaccine group has been suggested by some investigators.[31,62] Vaccine trials present an artificial situation whereby part of the herd remains unvaccinated and could potentially lead to fewer cases in nonvaccinated animals if protection is so effective that transmission of the pathogen is essentially shut down. However, the evidence for herd immunity from vaccinates suppressing the disease enough to reduce disease risk in the nonvaccinates is missing from the IBK field trials available. In published field trials,[31,60–63] the risk of IBK in vaccinated cattle is

consistently more than 25%, which is very similar to IBK levels seen in observational studies,[74] arguing against suppression and herd immunity as a realistic reason that field trials do not demonstrate efficacy.

- An insufficient sample size.[75,76] If null hypothesis significance testing is used to assess efficacy of a trial (ie, P values <.05 declared as significant effect), rather than the direction and precision of the effect size, then trials with insufficient sample size that used an effective vaccine might appear ineffective because of a type 2 error (the nonrejection of a false null hypothesis).[77] One solution would be to focus on interpretation of effect sizes and precision rather than P values. Often sample sizes are dependent on available research herds that give researchers the opportunity to examine eyes frequently, which is not always possible in commercial herds. Sample size calculations should therefore be included in reports to inform what power the study was able to achieve, that is, what the percent likelihood of being able to detect a difference between groups was. Field trials are also dependent on naturally occurring cases of IBK, and incidence can fluctuate from year to year. Sample sizes that rely on assumptions about expected incidence can therefore fall short if fewer cases occur than expected.

Although there are challenges in conducting vaccine trials under field conditions, they are the most reliable way to show that a vaccine will perform under similar conditions. The fact that there is such sparse evidence for vaccine efficacy in field trials is disappointing.

QUALITY ASSESSMENT OF VACCINE TRIAL STUDY DESIGN

During the initial experimental phase of vaccine development, challenge studies, which induce disease, use small numbers of animals in controlled environments. However, challenge studies are only a stepping stone in efficacy assessment because the controlled environment, disease model, or the challenge may all lead to low external validity. Although challenge studies are foundational and useful as a preliminary assessment for the potential of a new vaccine, the results are not necessarily indicative of how a vaccine will perform under field conditions. The blinded, randomized, placebo-controlled trial in the field with naturally occurring disease is the study design reference standard to document that a vaccine can protect a herd of cattle from IBK. Furthermore, to document that the results are repeatable, multiple trials conducted on multiple herds are required to truly assess the efficacy of a vaccine. When evaluating vaccine studies for IBK, criteria to assess the risk of bias should include assessment of the main risk domains confounding, selection bias, and information bias, as follows:

- Are the study groups comparable (exchangeable) with respect to all factors related to the outcome except the vaccine? Randomization is the process of chance allocation of study animals to treatment groups. If the sample size is sufficient, it reduces the potential for confounding of the results by other factors related to the outcome of interest, such as the age of animals.
- Is there a valid parallel comparator? In IBK vaccine trials, as there is no known effective vaccine, the use of a placebo control reduces the risk of differential treatment of groups and exposes all study animals to the same handling procedures and treatments except for the exposure to the vaccine antigen. Given the seasonality in IBK, the use of historic controls for IBK trials is invalid, as it is impossible to conclude that disease occurrence in a past year is representative of the expected disease experience in subsequent years. Use of a parallel comparator therefore controls the potential for selection bias.

- Are study personnel unaware of the treatment received? Blinding of outcome assessment reduces the potential for differential information bias. Blinded individuals should include those giving the treatments, those observing or caring for the animals, those assessing the outcome, and those performing the data analysis.
- Was a case definition or outcome parameter clearly stated a priori? Ensuring a clear repeatable outcome definition also reduces the potential for differential information bias. Although the definition of a case may be imperfect, it is most important that it does not differ for vaccinates and nonvaccinates.
- Are there losses to follow-up? It is essential that all animals enrolled in the trial are accounted for at the end of the trial. This is rarely an issue in IBK trials; however, it might be if young calves die because of concurrent diseases, such as respiratory disease or diarrhea. Uneven loss of animals from trials is associated with selection bias.

There is a trend toward reduced vaccine efficacy in trials that describe a higher number of important study design features (study population, vaccination regimen, placebo or adjuvant as the control group, clear case definitions, frequency and duration of disease assessment, randomization or blocking of treatment groups, blinding). Furthermore, only 20% (3/15) of trials that report randomization and blinding showed vaccine efficacy, compared with 43% (53) of all trials in a group of 123 trials conducted between 1960 and 2005, underlining that study design quality may be predictive of the direction of findings.[66]

OUTCOME METRICS FOR FIELD TRIALS

Studies on vaccine efficacy can also be compared by the measured outcomes. Is it more important to prevent clinical disease or is it enough to reduce severity or time to healing? Is a secondary outcome, such as weight gain, during the observation period or at some other predefined endpoint, such as at weaning, important for a cost-benefit analysis or as confirmation of findings from an imperfect case definition? Examples of group level outcomes that can be used to compare groups for IBK vaccine studies and possible caveats are as follows:

- Cumulative incidence, that is, the proportion in each group (vaccinated or unvaccinated) that developed IBK during the study period[31,60,61,63]
- Clinical score distribution; is the scoring system repeatable, reproducible, and validated?[30,78]
- Mean days to first ulcer[25,30]
- Mean or peak ulcer area for first ulcer; requires frequent observations[25]
- Proportion of those requiring treatment; was the threshold for treatment clearly stated[25]?
- Proportion of cases requiring multiple treatments; were criteria for giving multiple treatments stated[25]?
- Mean weaning weights or weight change during the study period[60,61,63]

SUMMARY

Despite 60 years of research into IBK vaccines, no effective vaccines appear to be widely available. We have gained understanding of the immunology surrounding IBK and antigenic nature of *M bovis* and other pathogens, but despite much effort, the factors needed to develop an effective vaccine remain elusive. IBK is multifactorial and is best explained by the epidemiologic triad of disease, which includes the host, the pathogen, and the environment that all contribute to disease outcome. From the available research, it appears that some challenge studies have suggested that vaccination could be effective when all the components of the triad can be controlled, that is, hosts are similar, the pathogen is a known strain, and there is no confounding by environmental factors, such as fly burden, sunlight, dust, or plant awns. Translating any success observed in challenge studies to the field remains elusive. The long list of reasons for why vaccines may have failed in field trials demonstrates the complexity of IBK epidemiology. However, the continued impact of this disease on animal welfare underlines the need for continued efforts to prevent IBK.

CLINICS CARE POINTS

- To date, there is no evidence that vaccines against infectious bovine keratoconjunctivitis are effective in the field. Even the encouraging results from experimental studies appear to be biased by poor study design and publication bias. It is unclear therefore even if experimental studies have been positive.
- Well-executed reproducible evidence of efficacy from multiple farms should be available for producers and veterinarians to assess the magnitude of the protective effect of vaccines.
- Proper study design will allow confidence in the results.
- Given the frustrating nature of infectious bovine keratoconjunctivitis and absence of publicly available evidence of efficacy, veterinarians should conduct on-farm trials of infectious bovine keratoconjunctivitis vaccines to assess the product effect at producers' farms. Such an evidence-based approach would allow empirical evidence for vaccine use.

DISCLOSURE

The authors have no commercial or financial conflicts of interest or funding sources to declare.

REFERENCES

1. Angelos JA, Spinks PQ, Ball LM, et al. Moraxella bovoculi sp. nov., isolated from calves with infectious bovine keratoconjunctivitis. Int J Syst Evol Microbiol 2007; 57(Pt 4):789–95.
2. Annuar BO, Wilcox GE. Adherence of Moraxella bovis to cell cultures of bovine origin. Res Vet Sci 1985;39(2):241–6.
3. Brinton CC Jr. The structure, function, synthesis and genetic control of bacterial pili and a molecular model for DNA and RNA transport in gram negative bacteria. Trans N Y Acad Sci 1965;27(8):1003–54.
4. Moore LJ, Lepper AW. A unified serotyping scheme for Moraxella bovis. Vet Microbiol 1991;29(1):75–83.
5. Simpson CF, White FH, Sandhu TS. The structure of pili (fimbriae) of Moraxella bovis. Can J Comp Med 1976;40:1–4.
6. Chandler RL, Baptista PJ, Turfrey B. Studies on the pathogenicity of Moraxella bovis in relation to infectious bovine keratoconjunctivitis. J Comp Pathol 1979; 89(3):441–8.
7. Ruehl WW, Marrs CF, George L, et al. Infection rates, disease frequency, pilin gene rearrangement, and pilin expression in calves inoculated with Moraxella bovis pilin-specific isogenic variants. Am J Vet Res 1993;54(2):248–53.
8. Ruehl WW, Marrs C, Beard MK, et al. Q pili enhance the attachment of Moraxella bovis to bovine corneas in vitro. Mol Microbiol 1993;7(2):285–8.

9. Bovre K, Froholm LO. Variation of colony morphology reflecting fimbriation in Moraxella bovis and two reference strains of M. nonliquefaciens. Acta Pathol Microbiol Scand B Microbiol Immunol 1972;80(5):629–40.

10. Marrs CF, Ruehl WW, Schoolnik GK, et al. Pilin-gene phase variation of Moraxella bovis is caused by an inversion of the pilin genes. J Bacteriol 1988;170(7): 3032–9.

11. Pugh GW Jr, Hughes DE. Experimental production of infectious bovine keratoconjunctivitis: comparison of serological and immunological responses using pili fractions of Moraxella bovis. Can J Comp Med 1976;40(1):60–6.

12. Jayappa HG, Lehr C. Pathogenicity and immunogenicity of piliated and nonpiliated phases of Moraxella bovis in calves. Am J Vet Res 1986;47(10):2217–21.

13. Lehr C, Jayappa HG, Goodnow RA. Controlling bovine keratoconjunctivitis with a piliated Moraxella bovis bacterin. Vet Med 1985;80(9):96, 98-100.

14. Lepper AW. Vaccination against infectious bovine keratoconjunctivitis: protective efficacy and antibody response induced by pili of homologous and heterologous strains of Moraxella bovis. Aust Vet J 1988;65(10):310–6.

15. Lepper AW, Atwell JL, Lehrbach PR, et al. The protective efficacy of cloned Moraxella bovis pili in monovalent and multivalent vaccine formulations against experimentally induced infectious bovine keratoconjunctivitis (IBK). Vet Microbiol 1995;45(2–3):129–38.

16. Dhungyel O, Hunter J, Whittington R. Footrot vaccines and vaccination. Vaccine 2014;32(26):3139–46.

17. Schwartzkoff CL, Egerton JR, Stewart DJ, et al. The effects of antigenic competition on the efficacy of multivalent footrot vaccines. Aust Vet J 1993;70(4):123–6.

18. Raadsma HW, O'Meara TJ, Egerton JR, et al. Protective antibody titres and antigenic competition in multivalent Dichelobacter nodosus fimbrial vaccines using characterised rDNA antigens. Vet Immunol Immunopathol 1994;40(3):253–74.

19. Lepper AW, Moore LJ, Atwell JL, et al. The protective efficacy of pili from different strains of Moraxella bovis within the same serogroup against infectious bovine keratoconjunctivitis. Vet Microbiol 1992;32(2):177–87.

20. Lepper AW, Elleman TC, Hoyne PA, et al. A Moraxella bovis pili vaccine produced by recombinant DNA technology for the prevention of infectious bovine keratoconjunctivitis. Vet Microbiol 1993;36(1–2):175–83.

21. Beard MK, Moore LJ. Reproduction of bovine keratoconjunctivitis with a purified haemolytic and cytotoxic fraction of Moraxella bovis. Vet Microbiol 1994;42(1): 15–33.

22. Gray JT, Fedorka-Cray PJ, Rogers DG. Partial characterization of a Moraxella bovis cytolysin. Vet Microbiol 1995;43(2–3):183–96.

23. Kagonyera GM, George LW, Munn R. Cytopathic effects of Moraxella bovis on cultured bovine neutrophils and corneal epithelial cells. Am J Vet Res 1989; 50(1):10–7.

24. Pugh GW Jr, Hughes DE. Experimental bovine infectious keratoconjunctivitis caused by sunlamp irradiation and Moraxella bovis infection: correlation of hamolytic ability and pathogenicity. Am J Vet Res 1968;29(4):835–9.

25. Angelos JA, Hess JF, George LW. Prevention of naturally occurring infectious bovine keratoconjunctivitis with a recombinant Moraxella bovis cytotoxin-ISCOM matrix adjuvanted vaccine. Vaccine 2004;23(4):537.

26. Hoien-Dalen PS, Rosenbusch RF, Roth JA. Comparative characterization of the leukocidic and hemolytic activity of Moraxella bovis. Am J Vet Res 1990;51(2): 191–6.

27. Billson FM, Hodgson JL, Egerton JR, et al. A haemolytic cell-free preparation of Moraxella bovis confers protection against infectious bovine keratoconjunctivitis. FEMS Microbiol Lett 1994;124(1):69–73.
28. Ostle AG, Rosenbusch RF. Immunogenicity of Moraxella bovis hemolysin. Am J Vet Res 1985;46(5):1011–4.
29. Angelos JA, Ball LM. Relatedness of cytotoxins from geographically diverse isolates of Moraxella bovis. Vet Microbiol 2007;124(3–4):382–6.
30. George LW, Borrowman AJ, Angelos JA. Effectiveness of a cytolysin-enriched vaccine for protection of cattle against infectious bovine keratoconjunctivitis. Am J Vet Res 2005;66(1):136–42.
31. Angelos JA, Gohary KG, Ball LM, et al. Randomized controlled field trial to assess efficacy of a Moraxella bovis pilin-cytotoxin-Moraxella bovoculi cytotoxin subunit vaccine to prevent naturally occurring infectious bovine keratoconjunctivitis. Am J Vet Res 2012;73(10):1670–5.
32. Postma GC, Carfagnini JC, Minatel L. Moraxella bovis pathogenicity: an update. Comp Immunol Microbiol Infect Dis 2008;31(6):449–58.
33. Brown MH, Brightman AH, Fenwick BW, et al. Infectious bovine keratoconjunctivitis: a review. J Vet Intern Med 1998;12(4):259–66.
34. Pedersen KB. The origin of immunoglobulin-G in bovine tears. Acta Pathol Microbiol Scand B Microbiol Immunol 1973;81(2):245–52.
35. Nayar PS, Saunders JR. Infectious bovine keratoconjunctivitis II. Antibodies in lacrimal secretions of cattle naturally or experimentally infected with Moraxella bovis. Can J Comp Med 1975;39(1):32–40.
36. Arora AK, Killinger AH, Myers WL. Detection of Moraxella bovis antibodies in infectious bovine keratoconjunctivitis by a passive hemagglutination test. Am J Vet Res 1976;37(12):1489–92.
37. Killinger AH, Weisiger RM, Helper LC, et al. Detection of Moraxella bovis antibodies in the SIgA, IgG, and IgM classes of immunoglobulin in bovine lacrimal secretions by an indirect fluorescent antibody test. Am J Vet Res 1978;39(6):931–4.
38. Bishop B, Schurig GG, Troutt HF. Enzyme-linked immunosorbent assay for measurement of anti-Moraxella bovis antibodies. Am J Vet Res 1982;43(8):1443–5.
39. Smith PC, Greene WH, Allen JW. Antibodies related to resistance in bovine pinkeye. Calif Vet 1989;43(4):7.
40. Webber JJ, Selby LA. Effects of Moraxella bovis vaccination schedules on experimentally induced infectious bovine keratoconjunctivitis. Am J Vet Res 1981;42(7):1181–3.
41. Pugh GW Jr. Infectious bovine keratoconjunctivitis: subconjunctival administration of a Moraxella bovis pilus preparation enhances immunogenicity. Am J Vet Res 1985;46(4):811–5.
42. Davidson HJ, Stokka GL. A field trial of autogenous Moraxella bovis bacterin administered through either subcutaneous or subconjunctival injection on the development of keratoconjunctivitis in a beef herd. Can Vet J 2003;44(7):577–80.
43. Misiura M. Estimation of fimbrial vaccine effectiveness in protection against keratoconjunctivitis infectiosa in calves considering different routes of introducing vaccine antigene. Arch Vet Pol 1994;34(3–4):177–86.
44. Misiura M. Keratoconjunctivitis infectiosa in calves–attempt at elimination by active immunization. Arch Vet Pol 1994;34(3–4):187–94.
45. Zbrun MV, Zielinski GC, Piscitelli HC, et al. Evaluation of anti-Moraxella bovis pili immunoglobulin-A in tears following intranasal vaccination of cattle. Res Vet Sci 2012;93(1):183–9.

46. Angelos JA, Edman JM, Chigerwe M. Ocular immune responses in steers following intranasal vaccination with recombinant Moraxella bovis cytotoxin adjuvanted with polyacrylic acid. Clin Vaccin Immunol 2014;21(2):181–7.

47. Cullen JN, Lithio A, Seetharam AS, et al. Microbial community sequencing analysis of the calf eye microbiota and relationship to infectious bovine keratoconjunctivitis. Vet Microbiol 2017;207:267–79.

48. Powe TA, Nusbaum KE, Hoover TR, et al. Prevalence of nonclinical Moraxella bovis infections in bulls as determined by ocular culture and serum antibody titer. J Vet Diagn Invest 1992;4(1):78–9.

49. Hughes DE, Pugh GW. Experimentally induced infectious bovine keratoconjunctivitis: vaccination with nonviable Moraxella bovis culture. Am J Vet Res 1972; 33(12):2475–9.

50. Pugh GW Jr, McDonald TJ, Kopecky KE. Infectious bovine keratoconjunctivitis: effects of vaccination on Moraxella bovis carrier state in cattle. Am J Vet Res 1980;41(2):264–6.

51. Pugh GW Jr, Kopecky KE, Kvasnicka WG, et al. Infectious bovine keratoconjunctivitis in cattle vaccinated and medicated against Moraxella bovis before parturition. Am J Vet Res 1982;43(2):320–5.

52. Hughes DE, Pugh GW Jr. A five-year study of infectious bovine keratoconjunctivitis in a beef herd. J Am Vet Med Assoc 1970;157(4):443–51.

53. Allan J, Van Winden S. Randomised control trial comparing cypermethrin-based preparations in the prevention of infectious bovine keratoconjunctivitis in cattle. Animals 2020;10(2):184.

54. Webber JJ, Selby LA. Risk factors related to the prevalence of infectious bovine keratoconjunctivitis. J Am Vet Med Assoc 1981;179(8):823–6.

55. Slatter DH, Edwards ME, Hawkins CD, et al. A national survey of the occurrence of infectious bovine keratoconjunctivitis. Aust Vet J 1982;59(3):65–8.

56. Snowder GD, Van Vleck LD, Cundiff LV, et al. Genetic and environmental factors associated with incidence of infectious bovine keratoconjunctivitis in preweaned beef calves. J Anim Sci 2005;83(3):507–18.

57. Pugh GW Jr, McDonald TJ, Booth GD. Infectious bovine keratoconjunctivitis: influence of age on development of disease in vaccinated and nonvaccinated calves after exposure to Moraxella bovis. Am J Vet Res 1979;40(6):762–6.

58. Salih BA, Ostle AG, Rosenbusch RF. Vaccination of cattle with Mycoplasma bovoculi antigens: evidence for field immunity. Comp Immunol Microbiol Infect Dis 1987;10(2):109–16.

59. Smith PC, Blankenship T, Hoover TR, et al. Effectiveness of two commercial infectious bovine keratoconjunctivitis vaccines. Am J Vet Res 1990;51(7):1147–50.

60. Cullen JN, Engelken TJ, Cooper V, et al. Randomized blinded controlled trial to assess the association between a commercial vaccine against Moraxella bovis and the cumulative incidence of infectious bovine keratoconjunctivitis in beef calves. J Am Vet Med Assoc 2017;251(3):345–51.

61. O'Connor A, Cooper V, Censi L, et al. A 2-year randomized blinded controlled trial of a conditionally licensed Moraxella bovoculi vaccine to aid in prevention of infectious bovine keratoconjunctivitis in Angus beef calves. J Vet Intern Med 2019; 33(6):2786.

62. O'Connor AM, Brace S, Gould S, et al. A randomized clinical trial evaluating a farm-of-origin autogenous Moraxella bovis vaccine to control infectious bovine keratoconjunctivis (pinkeye) in beef cattle. J Vet Intern Med 2011;25(6):1447–53.

63. Funk L, O'Connor AM, Maroney M, et al. A randomized and blinded field trial to assess the efficacy of an autogenous vaccine to prevent naturally occurring

infectious bovine keratoconjunctivis (IBK) in beef calves. Vaccine 2009;27(34): 4585–90.

64. Arora AK, Killinger AH, Mansfield ME. Bacteriologic and vaccination studies in a field epizootic of infectious bovine keratoconjunctivitis in calves. Am J Vet Res 1976;37(7):803–5.

65. Hughes DE, Kohlmeier RH, Pugh GW Jr. Comparison of vaccination and treatment in controlling naturally occurring infectious bovine keratoconjunctivitis. Am J Vet Res 1979;40(2):241–4.

66. Burns MJ, O'Connor AM. Assessment of methodological quality and sources of variation in the magnitude of vaccine efficacy: a systematic review of studies from 1960 to 2005 reporting immunization with Moraxella bovis vaccines in young cattle. Vaccine 2008;26(2):144–52.

67. Loy JD, Brodersen BW. Moraxella spp. isolated from field outbreaks of infectious bovine keratoconjunctivitis: a retrospective study of case submissions from 2010 to 2013. J Vet Diagn Invest 2014;26(6):761–8.

68. O'Connor AM, Shen HG, Wang C, et al. Descriptive epidemiology of Moraxella bovis, Moraxella bovoculi and Moraxella ovis in beef calves with naturally occurring infectious bovine keratoconjunctivitis (Pinkeye). Vet Microbiol 2012;155(2–4): 374–80.

69. Angelos JA, Lane VM, Ball LM, et al. Recombinant Moraxella bovoculi cytotoxin-ISCOM matrix adjuvanted vaccine to prevent naturally occurring infectious bovine keratoconjunctivitis. Vet Res Commun 2010;34(3):229–39.

70. Hughes DE, Pugh GW Jr, Kohlmeier RH, G D Booth. Effects of vaccination with a Moraxella bovis bacterin on the subsequent development of signs of corneal disease and infection with M bovis in calves under natural environmental conditions. Am J Vet Res 1976;37(11):1291–5.

71. Shah RR, Hassett KJ, Brito LA. Overview of vaccine adjuvants: introduction, history, and current status. Methods Mol Biol 2017;1494:1–13.

72. Zimmermann P, Curtis N. Factors that influence the immune response to vaccination. Clin Microbiol Rev 2019;32(2). e00084-18.

73. McConnel CS, House JK. Infectious bovine keratoconjunctivitis vaccine development. Aust Vet J 2005;83(8):506–10.

74. Funk LD, Reecy JM, Wang C, et al. Associations between infectious bovine keratoconjunctivitis at weaning and ultrasongraphically measured body composition traits in yearling cattle. J Am Vet Med Assoc 2014;244(1):100–6.

75. Akobeng AK. Understanding type I and type II errors, statistical power and sample size. Acta Paediatr 2016;105(6):605–9.

76. Mascha EJ, Vetter TR. Significance, errors, power, and sample size: the blocking and tackling of statistics. Anesth Analg 2018;126(2):691–8.

77. Szucs D, Ioannidis JPA. When null hypothesis significance testing is unsuitable for research: a reassessment. Front Hum Neurosci 2017;11:390.

78. i Girolamo FA, Sabatini DJ, Fasan RA, et al. Evaluation of cytokines as adjuvants of infectious bovine keratoconjunctivitis vaccines. Vet Immunol Immunopathol 2012;145(1–2):563.

79. Arora AK, Killinger AH, Mansfield ME. Bacteriologic and vaccination studies in a field epizootic of infectious bovine keratoconjunctivitis in calves. Am J Vet Res 1976;37(7):803–5.

A Review of Global Prevalence and Economic Impacts of Infectious Bovine Keratoconjunctivitis

Elliott J. Dennis, PhD[a],*, Mac Kneipp, BVSc, MVS, MANZCVS[b]

KEYWORDS

- Bos indicus • Bos taurus • Cattle • Infectious bovine keratoconjunctivitis • Pinkeye
- Economic • Prevalence

KEY POINTS

- Country-level prevalence of IBK has only been reported for the United States, Australia, and New Zealand.
- Prevalence rates of IBK are estimated by geographic climate and region accounting for cattle breed and age.
- Estimated prevalence of IBK worldwide is 2.78% of all beef cattle.
- Historical economic impact assessments are available for the United States, Australia, and United Kingdom.
- Economic impacts are implied and small, attributed to lower calf weaning weights and treatment costs but do not account for all factors likely underestimating IBK's full impact.

INTRODUCTION

Livestock diseases can impose significant costs on society.[1] Infectious bovine keratoconjunctivitis (IBK), commonly referred to as pinkeye, reportedly occurs worldwide[2] as the most significant ocular disease of cattle,[3,4] but all may not be reporting on the same disease entity.[2,5] Furthermore, there is large variation in animal susceptibility that affects estimates of prevalence and subsequent economic impact assessments. With few countries reporting national statistics on IBK, it is likely one of the leading underreported or misreported cattle diseases worldwide.

Cattle producers need knowledge of economic impacts to efficiently allocate resources to manage and/or mitigate IBK disease impacts. These assessments rely on first knowing the biological and epidemiologic drivers that determine prevalence

[a] University of Nebraska-Lincoln, 208A Filley Hall, Lincoln, NE 68583-0922, USA; [b] Sydney School of Veterinary Science, The University of Sydney, Camden, NSW, Australia
* Corresponding author.
E-mail address: elliott.dennis@unl.edu

Vet Clin Food Anim 37 (2021) 355–369
https://doi.org/10.1016/j.cvfa.2021.03.010
0749-0720/21/© 2021 Elsevier Inc. All rights reserved.
vetfood.theclinics.com

within heterogeneous cattle populations. These prevalence estimates can then be combined with input and output market prices and cattle populations to obtain aggregate country-level economic impacts.

This article has several objectives. We summarize the available literature on IBK prevalence by country and major IBK risk factors. Lacking disease prevalence for many countries, we develop a standardized and quantitative indication of IBK prevalence by geographic region using gridded livestock data. Last, we describe the existing literature that has quantified the global economic impact of IBK and address potential challenges and shortcoming with current and future estimates.

LITERATURE REVIEW
Methods

We conducted a literature search that covered industry and country-level reports, published journal articles, reports, and technical manuals using the following methods:

1. Online searches:
    a. Searches were conducted for estimates of IBK prevalence using a variety of search terms on CABI, ProMED, JSTOR, Elsevier, and Google scholar.
    b. Searches were conducted for economic impact assessments using the search terms "IBK" or "Moraxella" or "keratoconjunctivitis" and "economic" or "cost" on CABI, ProMED, JSTOR, Elsevier, and Google scholar.
2. Experts in the field of IBK were asked to provide any other suitable publications.
3. References from identified papers were reviewed.
4. Other relevant publications from pharmaceutical companies were reviewed.

BIOLOGY OF INFECTIOUS BOVINE KERATOCONJUNCTIVITIS
History and Risk Factors

IBK has been reported since the 1800s,[6,7] and no significant area of the world appears free.[2,3,8] However, knowledge of disease epidemiology is incomplete[9] and IBK may be a nonspecific umbrella term encompassing many different eye diseases in cattle rather than a single disease entity.[5,10] *Moraxella bovis,* a gram-negative bacterium, is considered the primary causal organism of IBK,[1] but the disease appears multifactorial.[11,12] Differing definitions of IBK may be one reason why there are wide differences in reported and estimated prevalence rates.

IBK risk factors can be categorized in the epidemiology triad of agent(s), host, and environment, including *M bovis* and its characteristics,[13–23] other agents such as *Mycoplasma* spp that may themselves be causal agents,[24,25] or ancillary, allowing *M bovis* to persist and create disease.[11,26,27] Environment factors include fomites[28] and vectors, particularly flies,[29–33] feeding method and pasture conditions,[12,31,34–36] season,[37–42] exposure to dust, plant debris and pollen,[43] and wind.[39] Host factors include breed,[3,44,45] age,[3,42,46,47] immune response,[4,8,48–50] concurrent illness, nutrition and body condition score, and stressors.[51] All these combine to impact the relative prevalence, or lack thereof, within specific countries.

Species and Breed Affected

Cattle breed is a major risk factor for IBK.[42] IBK is most common in subspecies *Bos taurus* (Bos taurus, British or European breeds) whereas *Bos indicus* (Bos taurus indicus, Brahman, zebu) appear resistant to natural IBK infection.[2,3,42,45,52–58] An analysis of health records of 45,497 calves in the United States from 1983 to 2002 concluded incidence of IBK was related to age of calf, cattle breed, and seasonal life cycle of the face fly, with a peak in summer. Incidence ranged from 22.4% in Herefords to 1.3% in

Pinzgauers and averaged 6.5% overall. Of 9 purebred *B taurus* breeds analyzed, Herefords were most susceptible, with a maternal effect on IBK incidence (higher in Hereford × Angus compared with Angus × Hereford calves). Incidence was less in calves crossbred with tropically adapted breeds (*B indicus*).[42]

PREVALENCE OF INFECTIOUS BOVINE KERATOCONJUNCTIVITIS

Few countries have estimated the prevalence of IBK. These estimates tend to vary by country, time, age of cattle, and herd size, making it difficult to generalize across space and time. Further, varying IBK case definitions likely exacerbates these differences. In our review of the literature, we found prevalence estimates from the United States, Australia, and New Zealand (**Table 1**). The next section summarizes these studies.

United States

Prevalence of IBK appears high in the United States, particularly in calves and in cow-calf operations, with up to 45% of calves affected during summer in some herds.[73] Data are sparse, with most estimates coming from university research farms,[67,72] individual states,[3,54,68] or the US Department of Agriculture (USDA). Overall, prevalence estimates are inconsistent, ranging from 1.1%[69] to 57% to 98%.[72] Estimates of prevalence are generally lower in national surveys than state-level surveys. The largest study of 45,497 calf health records indicated an overall IBK prevalence of 6.5% overall.[42]

Australia

Prevalence of IBK in Australia ranges greatly and varies by age, breed,[55,60] geographic location,[45,56,62] and over time, from 10%[61] to 43%[60] in calves. Several studies have reported IBK prevalence nationwide. In a recent survey of beef producers, 94.1% (990/1052) had pinkeye between 2014 and 2018, and 35.5% (373/1051) reported it every year during this period.[56] These estimates were comparable to an earlier study, which found 81% of beef and dairy producers reported IBK between 1975 and 1979.[45] This suggests that the prevalence rate of IBK has not changed considerably over time. Prevalence rates have historically been reported using head-level health records. A recent study estimated prevalence levels from sales of popular medication between 2015 and 2018 and found rates of 10.6% (95% prediction interval [PI] 6.31–17.59).[63] These are higher than the estimated national IBK prevalence of 4.5% in cows and 10% in calves.[35,45]

New Zealand

The first reported prevalence rates were in 1974, when it was suggested IBK may have been introduced for the first time.[64,66] All prevalence estimates were published in approximately 1980, when it was estimated to be in 9% of beef and dairy herds[65] and higher in Hereford cattle.[64] There are reported spatial differences with a 23% prevalence rate in Hunterville's district herds and 28% of herds in the Gisborne district. Of cattle in affected herds, 18% were young (<=1 year old) and 10% were adult stock (>1 year old).[66]

GLOBAL ESTIMATE OF PREVALENCE
Categorizing Cattle and Countries

In the absence of published prevalence rates from other nations, we provide approximate estimate prevalence rates in every country in the world using risk factors known to impact IBK.

Table 1
Summary of studies of estimating infectious bovine keratoconjunctivitis prevalence, by country

Year(s)	Cattle Type	Incidence Rate (%)	Location	Notes	Author or Reference
Australia					
1967	Calves	>90% in some herds	Queensland	In some herds during summer	Spradbrow,[59] 1967
1977	Other/Total	96% of Shorthorns	North Queensland	3% of Shorthorns permanently blinded	Dodt,[55] 1977
1977	Other/Total	53% of Brahman X	North Queensland		Dodt,[55] 1977
1975–1979	Calves	10%	Australia-wide	Dairy and beef cattle	Slatter et al,[45] 1982
1975–1979	Adult	4.5%	Australia-wide	Dairy and beef cattle	Slatter et al,[45] 1982
1984–1986	Calves	43.1% in Hereford X weaned heifers	North Queensland		Burns et al,[60] 1988
1984–1986	Calves	21.4% in Simmental X weaned heifers	North Queensland		Burns et al,[60] 1988
1984–1986	Calves	7.2% in Afrikander-Hereford X weaned heifers	North Queensland		Burns et al,[60] 1988
2006	Calves	10% of <1 year old	Australia-wide	MLA Modeling	Sackett et al,[61] 2006
2015	Other/Total	2.5% in southern Australia	Southern Australia	MLA Modeling	Lane et al,[62] 2015
2015	Other/Total	0.6% in northern Australia	Northern Australia	MLA Modeling	Lane et al,[62] 2015
2018	Other/Total	10.6% of all cattle	Australia-wide	Estimated from sales of medications	Kneipp et al,[63] 2020
2018	Other/Total	Median 5.7%	Australia-wide	Beef producer survey	Kneipp et al,[56] 2020
2018	Other/Total	94.1% had IBK in herd in last 5 y	Australia-wide	Beef producer survey	Kneipp et al,[56] 2020
2018	Other/Total	35.5% IBK in herd every year in last 5 y	Australia-wide	Beef producer survey	Kneipp et al,[56] 2020

New Zealand					
1979	Adult	18%	Hereford beef	IBK in past 5 y	Harris et al,[64] 1980
1979	Other/Total	27.9% and 15.8%	Hereford beef	IBK in past 5 y	Harris et al,[64] 1980
1975–1979	Other/Total	10.7%	Beef and dairy	At least one episode	Corrin,[65] 1980
1980	Other/Total	23% of farms	Hunterville district		Sinclair,[66] 1982
1980	Other/Total	28% of farms	Gisborne district		Sinclair,[66] 1982
1980	Calves	18%	Hunterville and Gisborne district		Sinclair,[66] 1982
1980	Cows	10%	Hunterville and Gisborne district		Sinclair,[66] 1982
United States					
1962–1967	Calves	58%	Iowa	5-y study University herd	Hughes &Pugh,[67] 1970
1962–1967	Adult	16% cows	Iowa	5-y study University herd	Hughes &Pugh,[67] 1970
1972	Calves	Up to 45% in some herds	Dixon Springs University of Illinois	During summer	Arora et al,[68] 1976
1976	Calves	20% beef calves	United States-wide	Approximately 10M beef calves & 3M feedlot cattle p.a.	USDA,[69] 1997; Hansen,[70] 2001
1976	Other	10% feedlot cattle	United States-wide	Approximately 10M beef calves & 3M feedlot cattle p.a.	USDA,[69] 1997; Hansen,[70] 2001
1978	Other/Total	8.75% in herds with endemic IBK	Missouri		Webber & Selby,[54] 1981
1978	Other/Total	45.4 reported endemic IBK	Missouri		Webber & Selby,[54] 1981
1993			Kansas	Second most common disease in cattle herds	Brown et al,[3] 1998
1996	Calves	11.3% of >3 wk old 0.6% of <3 wk	United States-wide	2700 beef producers surveyed	USDA,[69] 1997

(continued on next page)

Table 1
(continued)

Year(s)	Cattle Type	Incidence Rate (%)	Location	Notes	Author or Reference
1996	Adults	1.3% of all heifers and cows	United States-wide	2700 beef producers surveyed	USDA,[69] 1997
1996	Others	16.9% of all beef operations affected	United States-wide	2700 beef producers surveyed	USDA,[69] 1997
1996	Calves	1.1% ± 0.1 of unweaned calves > 3 wk old	United States-wide	Second most prevalent disease	USDA,[69] 1997
2007	Calves	2.2% of weaned calves treated with antibiotics	United States-wide		USDA,[71] 2010
2007	Adults	0.9% of cows treated with antibiotics	United States-wide		USDA,[71] 2010
2007	Adults	1.8% of cows culled due to bad eyes	United States-wide		
2007	Other/Total	2.1% of replacement heifers treated with antibiotics	United States-wide		USDA,[71] 2010
N/A	Calves	57%–98% yearlings per annum	UC Davis Field Station, California		Townsend,[72] 2013

Abbreviation: MLA, Meat and Livestock Australia.
Source: Author compiled.

Cattle breed, age, and geographic climate were identified as the most important risk factors affecting IBK prevalence. Cattle breed is the first primary risk factor for IBK. We divided domesticated cattle worldwide into 2 subspecies: (1) *B indicus,* which are adapted to hot climates, better able to use low planes of nutrition, and exhibit higher resistance to ticks, internal parasites, heat stress, and eye disease including IBK; and (2) *B taurus,* which are adapted to cooler climates, include almost all cattle breeds originating from Europe, and are more prone to IBK.[57,58] If uncertain, we categorized cattle on phenotype rather than strictly genotype. For example, Caribbean Senepol were classified *B indicus.*

Breed and geographic climate are highly correlated because breeds are adapted to thrive in certain climates. We assigned each global country to 1 of 3 different geographic climates: tropical, subtropical, and other. A country was tropical if the latitude of geographic centroid of the county lay between $-25° \leq x \leq 25°$, subtropical if between $-35° < x < -25°$ or $25° > x > 35°$, and other if between $-35° \leq x$ or $x \geq 35$. Cattle inventory within the country were then assigned a certain share of *B indicus* and *B taurus* cattle using published literature and expert opinion. The average [min, max] *B indicus* shares within a given climate are 0.95 [0.90, 1.00] in tropical, 0.20 [0.10, 0.30] in subtropical, and 0.05 [0.00, 0.10] in other. A triangle distribution is assumed across all climates.

Age is the third primary risk factor of IBK. We classify cattle as either cows (>1 year old) or calves (<=1 year old). No global estimates exist on the share of cows and calves within each country by cattle breed. We assume *B taurus* cattle are raised in more confined areas where culling unproductive cows is more common. Thus, we assume the share of cows within the *B taurus* cattle population to be 0.70 [0.60, 0.80]. The share of *B taurus* calves is 1 minus *B taurus* cows. Similarly, *B indicus* cattle are more commonly raised in larger areas where culling is less frequent. Thus, we assume the share of cows in the *B indicus* cattle population to be 0.80 [0.70, 0.90]. The share of *B indicus* calves is 1 minus *B indicus* cows. A triangle distribution is assumed across all cow and calf populations.

Average Prevalence Rates

Categorizing cattle by breed allows us to use published information on IBK prevalence rates. Rates from the United States, New Zealand, and Southern Australia are used to inform prevalence rates for *B taurus* cattle. From reported estimates in **Table 1**, we assume *B taurus* cows in a country's cattle population have an average annual IBK prevalence rate of 0.03 [0.01, 0.05] per annum. *B taurus* calves have an average prevalence rate of 0.10 [0.05, 0.20] per annum. Northern Australia is used to inform prevalence rates for *B indicus* cattle. From reported estimates in **Table 1**, we assume *B indicus* cows in a country's cattle population have an average annual prevalence rate of 0.006 [0.000, 0.020] per annum. *B indicus* calves have an average prevalence rate of 0.02 [0.01, 0.05] per annum.

Estimated Global Prevalence Rates

IBK prevalence rates by cattle breed are calculated as a weighted average of prevalence by cattle age. Estimated average prevalence rates are 0.88% [0.30, 2.30] for *B indicus* and 5.10% [2.60, 8.00] for *B taurus* cattle. Average prevalence rates within a given region is calculated as a weighted average of cattle breed and share of breeds in each geographic climate. Prevalence rate for cattle in tropical countries is 1.09% [0.53, 2.30], 4.26% [2.37, 6.29] for subtropical countries, and 4.89% [2.60, 7.43] for other countries. Prevalence rates are also aggregated by geographic region. These estimates together with other prevalence rates are reported in **Table 2**. Average

Table 2
Estimated number of cases, prevalence rate, and relative share of disease incidence

	Mode, %	Minimum, %	Maximum, %	Assumptions
Bos indicus				
Cow	0.60	0.00	2.00	
Calf	2.00	1.00	5.00	
Average	0.88	0.30	2.30	Assumes total cattle inventory has 0.8 [0.7, 0.9] share of cows; calf = 1 − cows
Bos taurus				
Cow	3.00	1.00	5.00	
Calf	10.00	5.00	20.00	
Average	5.10	2.60	8.00	Assumes total cattle inventory has 0.7 [0.6, 0.8] share of cows; calf = 1 − cows
Geographic climate				
Tropical	1.09	0.53	2.30	95% of live cattle inventory are *Bos indicus* breed, 5% are *Bos taurus*
Subtropical	4.26	2.37	6.29	20% of live cattle inventory are *Bos indicus* breed, 80% are *Bos taurus*
Other	4.89	2.60	7.43	5% of live cattle inventory are *Bos indicus* breed, 95% are *Bos taurus*
Region				Share of total countries in (Tropical, Subtropical, Other) climates
North America	4.73	2.54	7.15	(0, 25, 75)
Latin America and Caribbean	1.71	0.88	3.10	(82, 10, 8)
Europe and Central Asia	4.88	2.60	7.41	(0, 2, 98)
Middle East and North Africa	3.88	2.14	5.85	(14, 77, 9)
Sub-Saharan Africa	1.28	0.64	2.53	(94, 6, 0)
South Asia	3.69	2.01	5.66	(22, 56, 22)
East Asia and Pacific	1.90	0.98	3.37	(78, 8, 15)
Worldwide	2.78	1.66	4.00	(53, 16, 32)

Source: Authors' calculations.

prevalence rate worldwide is calculated as a weighted average of countries in each geographic climate. Estimated prevalence rate for cattle worldwide is 2.78% [1.66, 4.00].

GLOBAL ECONOMIC IMPACT
Previous Estimates of Economic Impact

It is frequently stated that IBK is the most costly ocular disease of cattle worldwide.[3,18,72] Empirical data quantifying these impacts are often lacking. In our review of the literature, only the United States, Australia, and the United Kingdom have published estimates on economic impacts. Most studies claiming large economic impacts infer these based on reduced weaning weights in calves. Rarely are impacts estimated at their true economic costs capturing actual losses in output, resources, prevention, and treatment efforts. We summarize all available studies in **Table 3**.

United States
The USDA (1976) estimated an annual loss of at least of $226 million.[70] Estimated costs ranged from $25 to $82 per head. No estimates accounted for impact of IBK to cows or other breeding livestock. Estimate was based on producer-reported treatment rates of pinkeye. Other reported studies calculated damages based on reduced weaning weight in calves multiplied by an average market price.

Australia
Australia conducted the first and most recent national economic impacts of IBK. The most frequently cited study quantifying the economic impacts of IBK remains a targeted postal survey of Australian beef and dairy producers in 1979.[45] Estimates were calculated by multiplying calculated prevalence rates, estimated loss per animal, and size of national herd. The estimated loss due to IBK in Australia was $15,140,000 in 1978, adjusted to $22,166,000 in 1982. This estimate did not account for cost of labor in treatment. Two subsequent studies sponsored by Meat and Livestock Australia modeled the impact of IBK to rank it against other red meat industry diseases. Estimates were AUS$23.2 million in 2006[61] and AUS$13.3 million in 2015.[62] However, given gross expenditure on 3 popular pinkeye medications alone was $9,670,000 each year from 2015 to 2018,[63] both appear to underestimate the full economic impact of IBK.

United Kingdom
The only study to estimate the economic impact of IBK in the United Kingdom was done in 1996.[76] Estimated cost due to IBK was $3.9 to $10.4 million per year. However, the study used IBK prevalence rates from the United States IBK, as there was a lack of available published literature. The estimate accounted for losses in output/resources, treatment costs, and prevention costs.

Alternative Global Estimates

Most studies examined either do not examine the full economic cost of IBK or estimate impacts on specific cattle subpopulations. The total economic cost of IBK could be separated into 4 components: direct losses to output, indirect losses to output, losses due to disease treatment, and losses due to disease prevention. Ideally, these costs should be estimated for relevant cattle subpopulations. Cattle breed, age, and geographic climate were 3 of the major risk factors we identified to estimate climate, region, and global prevalence rates of IBK. Estimating the economic cost components for each risk factor combination is one method that would capture the heterogeneity in IBK prevalence rates and full economic costs.

Table 3
Economic impact studies of bovine keratoconjunctivitis

Year	Economic Impact Total ($ mil)	Per Head ($/head)	Analysis	Notes	Author or Reference
United States					
1972–1975		25.76, 81.96	Used the reduction in weaning weight times average selling price of $40/cwt	For pinkeye in one and both eyes, respectively. Focused on reduction in weaning weight in calves+.	Killinger,[74] 1977
1975		60.58	Reduced weaning weight times $38/cwt	Can vary by breed (Hereford or Angus). Focused on reduction in weaning weight in calves.	Cobb et al,[75] 1976
2000	> 226.41			Used USDA-NAHMS results for calves and feedlot cattle.	Hansen et al,[70] 2001
Australia					
1979	16.7	9.51	Related prevalence in herds to estimate loss per affected animals and size of national herd	Based on producer estimates of economic cost. Included labor charges. Per estimates is a weighted average of estimates annual losses per head; treatment costs were estimated using treatment time, duration, and hourly cost.	Slatter et al,[45] 1982
2006	23.2			Australia-wide	Sackett et al,[61] 2006
2015	13.3	0.78		Southern herds	Lane et al,[62] 2015
2015		0.78		Northern herds	Lane et al,[62] 2015
2015	9.7			Used sales data as an indicator of IBK prevalence; likely lower bounds as did not account for labor and other costs associated with treatments.	Kneipp et al,[63] 2020
2015	6.9			(95% PI: 8.56, 13.11)	Kneipp et al,[63] 2020
United Kingdom					
1996	3.9–10.4			Incidence range derived from United States.	Bennett,[76,77] 2003

Abbreviations: NAHMS, National Animal Health Monitoring System; PI, prediction interval; USDA, US, Department of Agriculture.
Source: Author compiled.

SUMMARY AND IMPLICATIONS

Despite being reported for more than 130 years as the most significant ocular disease of any domestic species worldwide, prevalence rates and associated economic costs of IBK remain unclear. Prevalence rates tend to vary by country, time, age of cattle, and herd size, making it difficult to generalize across space and time. Reported rates come largely from producer surveys or university herds. There are likely differences in the definitions used to calculate prevalence rates, given that rates calculated from producer surveys are generally smaller than those from university herds. This would confirm some published reports that IBK is a nonspecific umbrella term encompassing many different eye diseases in cattle rather than a single disease entity.

Accurate economic assessments rely on combining known biological and epidemiologic drivers with market prices for inputs and outputs. This is particularly challenging for IBK because the basic biological knowledge is not settled. This is highlighted by the fact that there is not a single case definition for IBK. Furthermore, in most countries there are insufficient data to assess disease impacts, with only a modicum of biological and epidemiologic information available from the United States and Australia. Better data are required to properly estimate the global economic impact of IBK. In the absence of such data, inputs into economic models are likely to rely on expert opinion. Because economic estimates are used to inform the development of management alternatives with the potential role of private or government intervention, proper calibration of these economic parameters is paramount.

CLINICS CARE POINTS

- The prevalence of IBK varies. Evidence-based risk factors for IBK incidence include climate, cattle breed and age.
- Clinically significant disease is more prevalent in young, British and European breed cattle in warmer seasons.
- Clinicians should be wary of labeling outbreaks of ocular disease as IBK in adult Brahman cattle in mid-winter.

DISCLOSURE

The authors have nothing to disclose.

REFERENCES

1. Gould S, Dewell R, Tofflemire K, et al. Randomized blinded challenge study to assess association between *Moraxella bovoculi* and infectious bovine keratoconjunctivitis in dairy calves. Vet Microbiol 2013;164:108–15.
2. Wilcox GE. Infectious bovine kerato-conjunctivitis: a review. Vet Bull 1968;38:349–60.
3. Brown MH, Brightman AH, Fenwick BW, et al. Infectious bovine keratoconjunctivitis: a review. J Vet Intern Med 1998;12:259–66.
4. Postma GC, Carfagnini JC, Minatel L. *Moraxella bovis* pathogenicity: an update. Comp Immunol Microbiol Infect Dis 2008;31:449–58.
5. Aikman JG, Allan EM, Selman IE. Experimental production of infectious bovine keratoconjunctivitis. Vet Rec 1985;117:234–9.

6. Billings F. Keratitis contagiosa in cattle. Bull Agric Exp Station Nebr 1889;3: 247–52.

7. Penberthy JE. Contagious ophthalmia in cattle. J Compend Pathol Ther 1897;10: 263–4.

8. Baptista PJHP. Infectious bovine keratoconjunctivitis: a review. Br Vet J 1979;135: 225–42.

9. Cullen JN, Engelken TJ, Cooper V, et al. Randomized blinded controlled trial to assess the association between a commercial vaccine against Moraxella bovis and the cumulative incidence of infectious bovine keratoconjunctivitis in beef calves. J Am Vet Med Assoc 2017;251:345–51.

10. Punch PI, Slatter DH. A review of infectious bovine keratoconjunctivitis. Vet Bull 1984;54:193–207.

11. Schnee C, Heller M, Schubert E, et al. Point prevalence of infection with *Mycoplasma bovoculi* and *Moraxella* spp. in cattle at different stages of infectious bovine keratoconjunctivitis. Vet J 2015;203:92–6.

12. Alexander D. Infectious bovine keratoconjunctivitis: a review of cases in clinical practice. Vet Clin North America 2010;26:487–503.

13. Ruehl WW, Marrs CF, Fernandez R, et al. Purification, characterization, and pathogenicity of *Moraxella bovis* pili. J Exp Med 1988;168:983–1002.

14. Chandler RL, Baptista PJHP, Turfrey BA. Studies on the pathogenicity of *Moraxella bovis* in relation to infectious bovine keratoconjunctivitis. J Comp Pathol 1979; 89:441–8.

15. Annuar BO, Wilcox GE. Adherence of *Moraxella bovis* to cell cultures of bovine origin. Res Vet Sci 1985;62:1222–8.

16. Kopecky KE, Pugh GW, McDonald TJ. Infectious bovine keratoconjunctivitis: evidence for general immunity. Am J Vet Res 1983;44:260–2.

17. Pugh GW, Hughes DE. Comparison of virulence of various strains of *Moraxella bovis*. Can J Comp Med 1970;34:333–40.

18. Prieto C, Serra DO, Martina P, et al. Evaluation of biofilm-forming capacity of *Moraxella bovis*, the primary causative agent of infectious bovine keratoconjuntivitis. Vet Microbiol 2013;166:504–15.

19. Ostle AG, Rosenbusch RF. Immunogenicity of *Moraxella bovis* hemolysin. Am J Vet Res 1985;46:1011–4.

20. Beard MKM, Moore LJ. Reproduction of bovine keratoconjunctivitis with a purified haemolytic and cytotoxic fraction of *Moraxella bovis*. Vet Microbiol 1994;42: 15–33.

21. Farias LDa, Maboni G, Matter LB, et al. Phylogenetic analysis and genetic diversity of 3′ region of rtxA gene from geographically diverse strains of *Moraxella bovis*, *Moraxella bovoculi* and *Moraxella ovis*. Vet Microbiol 2015;178:283–7.

22. Angelos JA. Infectious bovine keratoconjunctivitis (pinkeye). Vet Clin North Am Food Anim Pract 2015;31:61–79.

23. Wilcox GE. The aetiology of infectious bovine keratoconjunctivitis in Queensland. 1. *Moraxella bovis*. Aust Vet J 1970;46:409–14.

24. Nayar PS, Saunders JR. Infectious bovine keratoconjunctivitis I. Experimental production. Can J Comp Med 1975;39:22–31.

25. Levisohn S, Garazi S, Gerchman I, et al. Diagnosis of a mixed mycoplasma infection associated with a severe outbreak of bovine pinkeye in young calves. J Vet Diagn Invest 2004;16:579–81.

26. Pugh GW, Hughes DE, Schultz VD. Infectious bovine keratoconjunctivitis: experimental induction of infection in calves with mycoplasmas and Moraxella bovis. Am J Vet Res 1976;37:57.

27. Rosenbusch RF. Influence of *Mycoplasma* pre-infection on the expression of *Moraxella* pathogenicity. Am J Vet Res 1983;44:1621–4.

28. Gelatt KN, Plummer CE. Color atlas of veterinary ophthalmology. 2nd edition. Ames, Iowa: Chichester, West Sussex: John Wiley & Sons, Inc; 2017.

29. Gerhardt RR, Allen JW, Greene WH, et al. The role of face flies in an episode of infectious bovine keratoconjunctivitis. J Am Vet Med Assoc 1982;180:156–9.

30. Berkebile D, Hall R, Webber J. Field association of female face flies with *Moraxella bovis*, an etiological agent of bovine pinkeye. J Econ Entomol 1981;74:475–7.

31. Hall RD. Relationship of the Face Fly (Diptera: Muscidae) to pinkeye in cattle: a review and synthesis of the relevant literature12. J Med Entomol 1984;21:361–5.

32. Shugart JI, Campbell DB, Hudson DB, et al. Ability of face fly to cause damage to eyes of cattle. J Econ Entomol 1979;72:633–5.

33. Brown J, Adkins T. Relationship of feeding activity of face fly (*Musca autumnalis* De Geer) to production of keratoconjunctivitis in calves. Am J Vet Res 1972;33: 2551–5.

34. Thrift F, Overfield J. Impact of pinkeye (infectious kerato-conjunctivitis) on weaning and postweaning performance of Hereford calves. J Anim Sci 1974;38: 1179–84.

35. Slatter DH, Edwards ME, Hawkins CD, et al. A national survey of the clinical features, treatment and importance of infectious bovine keratoconjunctivitis. Aust Vet J 1982;59:69–72.

36. Hughes DE. Infectious keratoconjunctivitis. In: Ristic M, McIntyre I, editors. Diseases of cattle in the tropics: economic and zoonotic relevance. Boston: M. Nijhoff Publishers; 1981. p. 237–45.

37. Kopecky KE, Pugh JGW, McDonald TJ. Influence of outdoor winter environment on the course of infectious bovine keratoconjunctivitis. Am J Vet Res 1981;42.

38. Pugh GW, Hughes DE. Bovine infectious keratoconjunctivitis: *Moraxella bovis* as the sole etiologic agent in a winter epizootic. J Am Vet Med Assoc 1972;161: 481–6.

39. Lepper AWD, Barton IJ. Infectious bovine keratoconjunctivitis: seasonal variation in cultural, biochemical and immunoreactive properties of Moraxella bovis isolated from the eyes of cattle. Aust Vet J 1987;64:33–9.

40. Cox P, Liddell J, Mattinson A. Infectious bovine keratoconjunctivitis: isolation of *Moraxella bovis* from two groups of young beef cattle in fly control field trials during 1981. Vet Rec 1984;115:29–32.

41. Wilcox GE. Bacterial flora of the bovine eye with special reference to *Moraxella* and *Neisseria*. Aust Vet J 1970;46:253–6.

42. Snowder GD, Van Vleck LD, Cundiff LV, et al. Genetic and environmental factors associated with incidence of infectious bovine keratoconjunctivitis in preweaned beef calves. J Anim Sci 2005;83:507–18.

43. George LW. Clinical infectious bovine keraotconjunctivitis. Compend Contin Educ 1984;6:712–22.

44. Frisch JE. The relative incidence and effect of bovine infectious keratoconjunctivitis in *Bos indicus* and *Bos taurus* cattle. Anim Prod 1975;21:265–74.

45. Slatter DH, Edwards ME, Hawkins CD, et al. A national survey of the occurrence of infectious bovine keratoconjunctivitis. Aust Vet J 1982;59:65–8.

46. Smith PC, Blankenship T, Hoover TR, et al. Effectiveness of two commercial infectious bovine keratoconjunctivitis vaccines. Am J Vet Res 1990;51:1147–50.

47. Jayappa HG, McVey DS. Moraxella. In: McVey DS, Kennedy M, Chengappa MM, editors. Veterinary microbiology. 3rd edition. Hoboken, USA: John Wiley & Sons, Inc; 2013. p. 145–7.

48. Frank SK, Gerber JD. Hydrolytic enzymes of *Moraxella bovis*. J Clin Microbiol 1981;13:269–71.
49. Angelos JA. Moraxella. In: Gyles CL, Prescott JF, Songer JG, et al, editors. Pathogenesis of bacterial infections in animals. 4th edition. Online: Blackwell Publishers; 2010. p. 469–81.
50. Fenwick BW, Rider MA, Liang J, et al. Iron repressible outer membrane proteins of *Moraxella bovis* and demonstration of siderophore-like activity. Vet Microbiol 1996;48:315–24.
51. Pugh GW Jr, McDonald TJ. Identification of bovine carriers of *Moraxella bovis* by comparative cultural examinations of ocular and nasal secretions. Am J Vet Res 1986;47:2343–5.
52. Canham AS. Ophthalmia in cattle. Vet J 1923;79:389–96.
53. Jackson FC. Infectious keratoconjunctivitis of cattle. Am J Vet Res 1953;14:19–25.
54. Webber JJ, Selby LA. Risk factors related to the prevalence of infectious bovine keratoconjunctivitis. J Am Vet Med Assoc 1981;179:823–6.
55. Dodt RM. The prevalence of bovine keratoconjunctivitis in a beef cattle herd in North Eastern Queensland. Aust Vet J 1977;53:128–31.
56. Kneipp M, Govendir M, Laurence M, et al. A national survey of the occurrence and risk factors associated with pinkeye in Australian beef cattle 2020.
57. Parsonson I. The Australian ark: a history of domesticated animals in Australia. Parkville, Australia: CSIRO Publishing; 2000.
58. Cooke RF, Daigle CL, Moriel P, et al. Cattle adapted to tropical and subtropical environments: social, nutritional, and carcass quality considerations. J Anim Sci 2020;98:skaa014.
59. Spradbrow PB. A microbiological study of bovine conjunctivitis and keratoconjunctivitis. Aust Vet J 1967;43:55–8.
60. Burns BM, Howitt CJ, Esdale CR. Bovine infectious keratoconjuncitivitis in different cattle breeds. Proc Aust Soc Anim Prod 1988;17:150–3.
61. Sackett D, Holmes P, Abbott K, et al. Assessing the economic cost of endemic disease on the production of Australian beef cattle and sheep production. North Sydney: Meat and Livestock Australia Ltd; 2006.
62. Lane J, Jubb T, Shephard R, et al. Priority list of endemic diseases for the red meat industries 2015. Available at: daf.qld.gov.au.
63. Kneipp M, Govendir M, Laurence M, et al. Current incidence, treatment costs and seasonality of pinkeye in Australian cattle estimated from sales of three popular medications 2020. Preventative veterinary medicine, 105232.
64. Harris RE, Cooper BS, Steffert IJ, et al. A survey of bovine infectious keratitis (pinkeye) in beef cattle. New Zealand Vet J 1980;28:58–60.
65. Corrin KC. Pinkeye in cattle. In: Fisheries MoAa, editor. Charcteristics and national survey. Weilington, New Zealand: Media services, Ministry of Agriculture and Fisheries; 1980.
66. Sinclair JA. Epidemiological aspects of infectious bovine keratoconjunctivitis in New Zealand. *Veterinary science*. Palmerston North: Massey University, New Zealand; 1982. p. 142.
67. Hughes DE, Pugh GW. A five-year study of infectious bovine keratoconjunctivitis in a beef herd. J Am Vet Med Assoc 1970;157:443–51.
68. Arora A, Killinger A, Mansfield M. Bacteriologic and vaccination studies in a field epizootic of infectious bovine keratoconjunctivitis in calves. Am J Vet Res 1976;37:803–5.

69. USDA A, Veterinary Services. NAHMS beef '97 Part II: reference of 1997 beef cow-calf health & health management practices [PDF] 1997. Available at: http://www.aphis.usda.gov/vs/ceah/ncahs/nahms/beefcowcalf/beef97/bf97pt2. pdf. Accessed July 25, 2018.

70. Hansen R. New tools in the battle against pinkeye. In: Proceedings of Nevada livestock production annual update: 2001. Reno: University of Nevada; 2001. p. 5–8.

71. USDA A, Veterinary Services. NAHMS beef 2007–08, Part IV: reference of beef cow-calf management practices in the United States, 2007–2008 2010. Available at: INFO@aphis.usda.gov.

72. Townsend WM. Food & fibre-producing animal ophthalmology. In: Gelatt KN, editor. Essentials of veterinary ophthalmology. Wiley: ProQuest Ebook Central; 2013. p. 384–90.

73. Arora AK, Killinger AH, Mansfield ME. Bacteriologic and vaccination studies in a field epizootic of infectious bovine keratoconjunctivitis in calves. Am J Vet Res 1976;37:803–5.

74. Killinger AH. Economic impact of infectious bovine keratoconjunctivitis in beef calves. Vet Med Small Anim Clin 1977;1977:618–20.

75. Cobb AB, Frahm RR, Mizell RH. Effect of pinkeye on weaning weight of beef calves. In: Oklahoma state university research report. Oklahoma: Oklahoma State University; 1976. p. 61.

76. Bennett R. The 'direct costs' of livestock disease: the development of a system of models for the analysis of 30 endemic livestock diseases in Great Britain. J Agric Econ 2003;54:55–71.

77. Chaters G, Johnson P, Cleaveland S, et al. Analysing livestock network data for infectious disease control: an argument for routine data collection in emerging economies. Philos Trans R Soc B 2019;374:20180264.

Future Directions for Research in Infectious Bovine Keratoconjunctivitis

Annette M. O'Connor, BVSc, MVSc, DVSc, FANZCVS[a],*,
John A. Angelos, DVM, PhD, DACVIM[b], Elliott J. Dennis, PhD[c],
Paola Elizalde, DVM, MS[d], Mac Kneipp, BVSc, MVS, MANZCVS[e],
John Dustin Loy, DVM, PhD[f], Gabriele Maier, DVM, MPVM, PhD, DACVPM[g]

KEYWORDS

- Antibiotics • Infectious bovine keratoconjunctivitis • Research • Vaccination
- Pinkeye prevention

KEY POINTS

- Many unanswered questions remain about the epidemiology of infectious bovine kerato-conjunctivitis (IBK), especially the role of potential risk factors, such as other microorganisms besides *Moraxella bovis*, and nonmicrobial causes of IBK, such as flies.
- New study approaches that ask refined research questions with study designs that do not repeat older studies are needed to advance our knowledge of IBK; in particular, multilocation prospective studies would provide more information than cross-sectional studies.
- Research into modern, effective vaccines remains a priority despite the difficulties designing vaccines against bacterial pathogens living on mucosal surfaces.
- Research into alternative control approaches, such as fly control, is also needed.
- More research is needed to provide evidence for alternatives to antibiotics for treating IBK. No studies give information on the efficacy of these approaches, although they appear to be commonly used.

[a] Department of Large Animal Clinical Sciences, College of Veterinary Medicine, Michigan State University, East Lansing, MI, USA; [b] Department of Medicine and Epidemiology, School of Veterinary Medicine, University of California Davis, CA, USA; [c] Department of Agricultural Economics, Lincoln, NE, USA; [d] School of Public Health, University of Saskatchewan, Saskatoon, Saskatchewan, Canada; [e] Sydney School of Veterinary Science, The University of Sydney, Australia; [f] Nebraska Veterinary Diagnostic Center, School of Veterinary Medicine and Biomedical Sciences, University of Nebraska-Lincoln, Lincoln, NE, USA; [g] Department of Population Health & Reproduction, School of Veterinary Medicine, University of California Davis, CA, USA
* Corresponding author.
E-mail address: oconn445@msu.edu

Vet Clin Food Anim 37 (2021) 371–379
https://doi.org/10.1016/j.cvfa.2021.03.011
0749-0720/21/© 2021 Elsevier Inc. All rights reserved.

INTRODUCTION

In this issue of the *Veterinary Clinics of North America: Food Animal Practice*, the authors have focused on infectious bovine keratoconjunctivitis (IBK). The articles in this issue have looked at the diagnosis, epidemiology, and economic impact of IBK. The articles have also looked at the basis for, and effect of, interventions to treat or prevent IBK. This article discusses what remains unknown and why it matters that the research community focuses on helping producers solve IBK.

DIAGNOSIS

The diagnosis of IBK seems to be more contentious than one would be expecting. The article on this topic discusses the need for a clear case definition of the disease so that we know all researchers are studying the same disease and the use of standardized terminology, so reports are comparable. An unbiased, repeatable IBK score is also desirable for global cattle industries, so that lesions may be objectively described, for example, before sale and for quality assurance. As eyes respond to noxious challenge in a stereotypical manner, digital images combined with machine learning informed by standard ophthalmic descriptors show great potential for such an IBK score in the future. The clinical characteristics to allow for diagnosis of IBK in an individual and in a herd are described in the article on diagnosis, but these could be further refined by interest from veterinary ophthalmologists using their particular skillset. Some ophthalmic techniques could be further adapted for better use on cattle in the field, for example, fluorescein staining and Schirmer tear tests.

Recent advances in molecular biology-based techniques, such as polymerase chain reaction (PCR), offer the hope of point-of-care diagnosis of IBK both to detect and to differentiate between pathogens. PCR assay has been used to confirm a diagnosis of *M bovis*.[1] An IBK study found that PCR detected organisms from lacrimal fluid more frequently and reported more than 1 organism more often than culture.[2] A multiplex real-time PCR panel assay using 2 reactions was highly sensitive and highly specific for detection and differentiation of the 5 major pathogens associated with bovine ocular disease, *Moraxella bovis*, *Moraxella bovoculi*, *Mycoplasma bovis*, *Mycoplasma bovoculi*, and bovine herpesvirus type 1.[3] Ongoing efforts by the research community mean such tests should become more available and user-friendly in future.

EPIDEMIOLOGY

A full understanding of the epidemiology of IBK remains elusive. From the 3 articles devoted to component causes of IBK, it is evident that much remains to be understood. We do not fully understand why some herds have a high incidence of IBK and others a low incidence. Within herds, we do not know why some animals develop IBK and others do not.

The large ruminants appear uniquely prone to epidemic disease confined to the eye. Infectious keratoconjunctivitis (IKC) also occurs in sheep,[4] goats, and wildlife, such as ibex, chamois, and deer,[5] but in all species other than cattle, IKC is considered multifactorial in nature. The conventional bacterial paradigm of IBK with *M bovis* as a primary corneal pathogen is contrary to ophthalmologic principles of avoiding labeling corneal disease as "eye infection" when primary bacterial infection of the cornea "basically does not exist" and cultures are of not much value.[6]

Traditionally, we have thought of IBK as an infectious disease with *M bovis* as the causal agent. Indeed, there is evidence that *M bovis* is an important component cause of IBK. However, it is evident from reading the article on the component causes of IBK associated with *Moraxella* spp that we still do not understand the role of *M bovoculi*. The observational findings that *M bovoculi* is more commonly recovered from IBK lesions than *M bovis*, and that *M bovoculi* possesses toxins similar in structure and function to *M bovis* are not easily dismissed. However, we lack other evidence of a causal role, especially the absence of challenge model data, which are so commonly the primary source of causal evidence in veterinary science.

The research community should consider how we would either build a body of evidence for causation or how we can reach a conclusion that perhaps *M bovoculi* is not causal. We probably are at the point where we know that *M bovoculi* is more common in ocular lesions than *M bovis*. Repeating this finding will not add much to the evidence base. Instead, there is a need for studies that focus on differences in animals that develop IBK and those that do not. Such studies are likely to provide much more exact information about the characteristics of *M bovis* or *M bovoculi* that cause IBK. We also need to move beyond the simple classification of *M bovis* and *M bovoculi* and instead use more nuanced categories of *Moraxella* spp. This work has already begun with some of the recent molecular genomic work, and it is hoped it will provide some clarity about what is associated with virulence. For example, that both *M bovis* and *M bovoculi* genomes are dynamic and some demonstrate interspecies recombination, sometimes in known virulence factors such as toxins, makes assignment of many strains to a single species very challenging. There is also opportunity for the applications of genomics to the bovine host. As whole-genome sequencing is now available at the individual animal level, there are opportunities to link pathogen, disease, and host through association studies.

The article about non-Moraxella–associated component causes of IBK documents the lack of evidence about other component causes. For some of these agents, such as the Mycoplasmas, there have been significant technological developments that make studying these fastidious organisms possible. There also appear to be opportunities to better understand the epidemiology of IBK by studying these putative risk factors. However, the reason these factors, such as long grass, pasture species composition, UV light levels, and genetics, have not been so thoroughly studied may be because there seems to be little opportunity to manipulate these factors. Without an option to intervene, knowing that these factors are associated with IBK is informative, but not necessarily helpful.

On the other hand, the role of flies in the epidemiology of IBK remains an unexplored area where there is the potential for manipulation that could help with control. However, the study designs associated with evaluating if flies are causally related to IBK are challenging to conduct. It would be necessary to enroll a large number of farms and conduct either an ecological association or a hierarchical study that looks at the role of flies in the incidence of IBK at the herd level and the individual level. It is unclear why such studies have not been conducted to date, but the most probable reasons include the difficulty of organizing and funding multifarm studies.

Finally, another aspect of the epidemiology of IBK that seems dramatically underresearched is the issue of IBK in dairy herds. Very few studies have been conducted in modern dairy production systems; therefore, we simply do not know how dairy production impacts the epidemiology of IBK and how important IBK is in dairy calf production.

ECONOMIC IMPACT

The absence of high-quality surveys or production data about the incidence of IBK within and between herds is a glaring omission in the body of literature. The article on prevalence and impact of IBK points out that livestock diseases can impose substantial costs on society. Notwithstanding that IBK is the most important ocular disease of cattle worldwide, there are very little data available from the global community on the occurrence or industry losses it causes. These losses lead us to believe that it is likely one of the leading underreported or misreported cattle diseases worldwide. Correct economic impact estimates are required so government and private industry can allocate the optimal amount of research and development expenditures. These estimates provide an appropriate baseline where the tradeoffs between mitigation or treatment strategies can be evaluated.

Currently, we do not have adequate data that are up-to-date for beef production systems that describe how many herds and animals within herds have been or are likely to be impacted by IBK. Furthermore, there are almost no data about the impact of IBK in dairy production systems. A cursory review of the literature suggests that these impacts would likely be slightly larger than current impacts on the beef production system. Most of the data on economic impacts are based on individual trials from university herds whereby estimated weight loss at either weaning or postweaning is multiplied by market prices. Studies on the economic impacts are primarily from the United States and Australia. There is little to no information of IBK's impact in developing countries. This lack of information is particularly concerning given the role livestock plays as a store of wealth and food security. Likewise, developing countries have both different climates and cattle than Australia and United States, and thus likely different incidence rates and subsequent economic impacts. Although these estimates are thought to be smaller in magnitude, the relative impact is likely much greater.

The absence of information on economic impacts might be the most critical information we need as a research community if the desire to help veterinarians and producers prevent and control IBK. Regular surveillance and reporting on the prevalence and impact of IBK around the world are warranted if there is a desire by the international community to monitor the economic impacts over time. Looking at the example of bovine respiratory disease (BRD), every study appears to lead with the major rationale that BRD is the most economically important disease of cattle, and these estimates have remained a consistent theme over time. Although it is not likely that IBK would increase to the level of cost of BRD, continuing to argue the disease matters without economic data seems futile. The ideal data that would enable the most robust economic assessment of the real costs of IBK in beef and dairy production systems would originate from producers' historical health databases. These data would enable analyses of IBK over time by assessing how management and animal characteristics impact economic estimates. In the absence of this production-level data, surveys can serve as an appropriate substitute given proper survey instrument calibration and appropriate sample participants. In developing countries where production-level data may be lacking, this is likely the ideal first step to obtain economic impact estimates.

PREVENTION

A large amount of research in recent years on IBK has evaluated either novel or commercially available vaccination products. The work on commercially available vaccination products is surprisingly sparse and has shown no evidence that they are effective. Moreover, the work is limited in its scope to single locations. It would be far better if the evaluations of commercial vaccines were conducted at multiple sites over multiple years. Such information will help producers and veterinarians understand either the variability of vaccine responses (if it is shown that at some locations the vaccines are effective) or the consistency of vaccine responses (if it is shown that the vaccines consistently do not work). The value of studies conducted over the past 10 years may be the documentation of the need for more research into vaccine development.

Vaccines against *M bovis* or *M bovoculi* that are on the market are administered parenterally. Although this type of vaccine induces an immunoglobulin G (IgG) antibody response in serum, they seem to fail in inducing a local IgA antibody response in the eye. It is probably a reasonable assumption that development of vaccines that can be administered locally on the mucosal surface to enhance the production of protective IgA antibody against *Moraxella* spp will be important for protection against IBK associated with *Moraxella* spp; however, unequivocal proof that anti–Moraxella IgA in the eye equates to protection from disease is lacking. There is an essential need to develop new vaccines based on new technologies. Even if it were shown that current vaccines were effective in some locations but not others, it would still leave some producers and veterinarians with a product that does not work for them. At a minimum, reasons for vaccine failure, such as serogroup mismatch, should be explored and would require vaccine manufacturers to disclose serogroups of vaccine strains. Ideally, new vaccines developed using the latest technologies would have a consistent effect across all herds. A consistent effect is what we have come to expect from vaccines in human health. We do not generally expect vaccines, such as measles, mumps, rubella, and chickenpox, to work in some people and not in others. We should have the same expectation for IBK vaccines. Certainly, neither veterinary nor human vaccines are marketed as only working in a subgroup of the population of people or herds.

As we move forward with development of new vaccines, it will be critical that the US Department of Agriculture (USDA) Center for Veterinary Biologics makes publicly available the evidence of efficacy for any newly approved products. There is a movement toward having the USDA Center for Veterinary Biologics provide such information equivalent to that provided by the Food and Drug Administration Center for Veterinary Medicine in the Freedom of Information summaries for new antibiotics.

M bovis has demonstrated iron acquisition systems.[7] Lactoferrin is a component of the innate immune system that exerts bacteriostatic effects by depriving bacteria of iron and is found in high concentrations in many secretory fluids, including bovine tears.[8] Further characterization of the normal defense mechanisms of the bovine eye and how *M bovis* overcomes bacteriostatic lactoferrin in tears may lead to new strategies to enhance the immune response against *M bovis*.[8] Topical treatments targeting bacterial requirements for iron and vaccines to immunize against bacterial siderophores are promising research areas.[9] Research is needed to further our knowledge of the ocular microbiome in healthy and IBK affected eyes as well as the role that *Moraxella* spp biofilms may play at the bovine ocular surface.

As mentioned in the topic on the epidemiology of IBK, fly control may represent an area of intervention that has not been thoroughly investigated. The studies that were conducted many years ago on fly control were quite elegant. Repeating those studies with animals with new fly-control products should be considered. An alternative approach would be to conduct large-scale studies that somehow control for the potential cross-contamination of research groups that can occur in insecticide studies. The survey of fly-control products is always problematic because the most natural experimental unit is the herd. When the herd is the unit of concern, the sample size required can be enormous and beyond a single researcher's capacity. Ideally, we would allocate animals within herds to fly-control products, but we risk cross-contamination of the group that is not treated, which would nullify the results. However, a multistate collaboration could effectively address this issue. A team of researchers could enroll herds in their state, randomize within the group, and evaluate the incidence of IBK in treated versus untreated herds. The design could also have a crossover component. In 1 year, herds could be allocated randomly, and then the next year, the herds crossover to the other allocation. Such an approach would provide some control for herd-level effects.

The significant variation of IBK incidence between breeds has led to interest in IBK as a heritable trait and genetic selection for IBK resistance. A review of health records of 45,497 beef calves in the United States estimated the heritability of IBK incidence for all breeds was between 0.00 and 0.28.[10] A study of tropically adapted *Bos taurus* composite calves in Queensland concluded IBK is a heritable trait with low to moderate heritability of 0.17 to 0.19.[11] Two studies concluded heritability of IBK in Angus cattle in the United States was low, between 0.05 and 0.11[12] and 0.06 and 0.10.[13] Although IBK disease appears to be a lowly heritable complex trait that is polygenic in nature and subject to environmental effects, studies to discover any genetic markers associated with host resistance are warranted in the hope there may be incremental improvements in breed resistance to disease.

TREATMENT

Treatment of IBK currently relies on antibiotics and untested alternatives to antibiotics with unknown efficacy. There are gaps in our knowledge about IBK treatments. Even for the popular antibiotics used to treat IBK, there are few pharmacology studies available. For example, intramuscular oxytetracycline (OTC) is reported to be an effective treatment for IBK,[14,15] but how it works is unclear. Despite being an amphoteric molecule that should theoretically diffuse into tears, OTC was not detected in tears of treated animals.[14] Knowledge of the level of active drug at the site of infection, the surface of the eye, would be valuable. Pharmacokinetic profile studies of drugs in tears using high-performance liquid chromatography make this possible with a little research effort.

As an area of research, treatment options for IBK are not likely as impactful as randomized control trials for vaccine products. However, despite the difficulty of conducting treatment trials, 1 advantage is that the products of interest to be evaluated are readily available. As an alternative to injected antibiotics, some producers and veterinarians are using eye ointments, sprays, eye flaps, and patches. Therefore, research into efficacy of these modalities could be immediately informative to producers and veterinarians. Unlike vaccines, which require a great deal of preliminary data before field testing, commonly used IBK treatments could be more readily conducted.

These studies should also be conducted because we have 2 pressures to reduce our use of antibiotics, even for a disease such as IBK. First, as part of antibiotic stewardship, we would like to reduce the use of antibiotics, so knowledge of nonantibiotic treatment options and how they compare to antibiotics is important. This information can be used by organic producers and nonorganic producers in the overall effort to reduce antibiotic use. Prudent use of antimicrobial agents is a consideration in choice of IBK treatment with single-drug treatment preferable and use of multiple antibiotics not generally recommended for reasons of economy and good antimicrobial stewardship.[16] Producer education is also vital for preventing unnecessary administration of antibiotics to IBK-affected animals, especially once the disease has run its course and healing is well underway. With increased scrutiny of antimicrobial use in livestock, there is renewed interest in non-antimicrobials. *M bovis*[17] and *M bovoculi*[18] can form biofilms that may be important in the pathogenesis of ocular moraxellosis. Use of 10% magnesium chloride (MgCl$_2$) was described to inhibit autoagglutination of *M bovis* in liquid media[19] and may be useful for treatment of IBK.[17] Results from a randomized blinded challenge study involving 30 calves indicated hypochlorous acid may be used as alternative therapy to reduce pain, infection, and healing time of corneal lesions in calves experimentally infected with *M bovis*.[20] The need for non-antibiotic alternatives is a pressing concern, as *M bovoculi* strains with multidrug resistance have been described that are resistant to most antibiotics approved for treatment and were recently listed in the American Veterinary Medical Association's antimicrobial-resistant pathogens affecting animal health in the United States.[a]

There is also a surprising need to have information about the comparative efficacy of antibiotics registered for use. This information would enable producers and veterinarians to make informed choices about which antibiotic to use if an antibiotic will be used from a health perspective and efficacy.

It would be beneficial if such studies were planned with knowledge of intended use in a network meta-analysis. This knowledge would impact the referent group chosen and the outcome. In IBK research, we do not have an enormous amount of funding. Therefore, as a community, if researchers could more efficiently combine research from multiple researchers, we could leverage that information to know more. This process does not limit the outcomes that could be assessed. Researchers could assess any outcome of interest to them; the idea would be for the research community to agree to 1 or 2 common outcomes to be evaluated. The Core Outcome Measures in Effectiveness Trials (COMET) Project group is 1 approach to try to determine a standard set of outcomes. A community of researchers works together to maximize the value of the work being done. COMET is defined as "[a] core outcome set (COS) is an agreed standardized set of outcomes that should be measured and reported, as a minimum, in all clinical trials in specific areas of health or health care." Standardization of disease scoring rubrics and treatment decision thresholds could maximize knowledge obtained from using such an approach.

GENERAL PRINCIPLES

The IBK research community should also consider generally embracing newer concepts of science. New ideas, such as open access, sharing of datasets, open peer review, and a priori protocol publication, can increase the value of funding directed at IBK. Open access ensures that the information is available to anyone who seeks access to it. Sharing datasets enables reanalysis as new methods are developed and potentially enables patient-level meta-analysis, which is better for understanding individual-level confounding. Open peer review encourages the readers of a manuscript to find out concerns that reviewers may have. Researchers are often able to build better subsequent studies based on the critiques identified in open peer reviews. A priori protocol publication would reduce the potential for publication bias; thus, we would be aware of studies conducted but not published and have the opportunity to determine why the results are missing from the knowledge base. A priori protocol publication also increases the probability that studies will be published even if only in conference abstract format, which is better than entirely hidden.

---

[a] https://www.avma.org/sites/default/files/2020-10/AntimicrobialResistanceFullReport.pdf.

SUMMARY

In conclusion, although significant progress has been made over the years in IBK research, much remains unknown. The focus on vaccination will continue, as it should. However, effective bacterial vaccines remain elusive, and until new technologies, such as antigens that may be broadly protective and those that induce mucosal immunity, become available that increase the likelihood of success, it is worth pursuing other avenues. Particularly fruitful areas appear to be control, treatment options, and the economic costs of IBK. The resources available for IBK research are limited, but the community of researchers has done an amazing job leveraging small amounts of funding for maximum impact. It would be extremely impactful and also increase external validity if a worldwide community of IBK researchers with expertise in microbiology, genetics, genomics, diagnostics, vaccinology, epidemiology, and statistics could support each other in conducting studies.

DISCLOSURE

The authors have nothing to disclose.

REFERENCES

1. Loy DJ, Brodersen BW. *Moraxella spp.* isolated from field outbreaks of infectious bovine keratoconjunctivitis: a retrospective study of case submissions from 2010 to 2013. J Vet Diagn Invest 2014;26:761–8.
2. O'Connor AM, Shen HG, Wang C, et al. Descriptive epidemiology of Moraxella bovis, Moraxella bovoculi and Moraxella ovis in beef calves with naturally occurring infectious keratoconjunctivitis (pinkeye). Vet Microbiol 2012;155:374–80.
3. Zheng W, Porter E, Noll L, et al. A multiplex real-time PCR assay for the detection and differentiation of five bovine pinkeye pathogens. J Microbiol Methods 2019; 160:87–92.
4. Chapman HM, Murdoch FR, Robertson ID, et al. Detection, identification and treatment of infectious Ovine keratoconjunctivitis (Pink Eye) in sheep from a Western Australian pre-export feedlot. North Sydney: Meat & Livestock Australia; 2010.
5. Tryland M, Stubsjøen SM, Ågren E, et al. Herding conditions related to infectious keratoconjunctivitis in semi-domesticated reindeer: a questionnaire-based survey among reindeer herders. Acta Veterinaria Scand 2016;58(22):1–10.
6. Wilcock BP. General Pathology of the Eye. In: Maggs DJ, Miller PE, Ofri R, editors. Slatter's fundamentals of veterinary ophthalmology. 4th edition. St Louis (MO): Saunders Elsevier; 2008. p. 62–80.
7. Postma GC, Carfagnini JC, Minatel L. Moraxella bovis pathogenicity: an update. Comp Immunol Microbiol Infect Dis 2008;31:449–58.
8. Brown MH, Brightman AH, Fenwick BW, et al. Infectious bovine keratoconjunctivitis: a review. J Vet Intern Med 1998;12(4):259–66.
9. Sodhi N. Could immunisation be a key in the fight against bacterial resistance? Aust Vet J 2017;95(3):N8.
10. Snowder GD, Van Vleck LD, Cundiff LV, et al. Genetic and environmental factors associated with incidence of infectious bovine keratoconjunctivitis in preweaned beef calves. J Anim Sci 2005;83:507–18.
11. Ali AA, O'Neill CJ, Thomson PC, et al. Genetic parameters of infectious bovine keratoconjunctivitis and its relationship with weight and parasite infestations in Australian tropical *Bos taurus* cattle. Genet Selection Evol J 2012;44(22):1–10.

12. Rodriguez JE. Infectious bovine keratoconjunctivitis in Angus cattle. Ames: Iowa State University; 2006.
13. Kizilkaya K, Tait RG, Garrick DJ, et al. Genome-wide association study of infectious bovine keratoconjunctivitis in Angus cattle. BMC Genet 2013;14:23.
14. George LW, Smith JA, Kaswan R. Distribution of oxytetracycline into ocular tissues and tears of calves. J Vet Pharmacol Ther 1985;8:47–54.
15. George LW, Smith JA. Treatment of Moraxella bovis infections in calves using a long-acting oxytetracycline formulation. J Vet Pharmacol Ther 1985;8:55–61.
16. Angelos JA. Infectious bovine keratoconjunctivitis (pinkeye). Vet Clin North Am Food Anim Pract 2015;31:61–79.
17. Prieto C, Serra DO, Martina P, et al. Evaluation of biofilm-forming capacity of Moraxella bovis, the primary causative agent of infectious bovine keratoconjunctivitis. Vet Microbiol 2013;166:504–15.
18. Ely VL, Vargas AC, Costa MM, et al. Moraxella bovis, Moraxella ovis and Moraxella bovoculi: biofilm formation and lysozyme activity. J Appl Microbiol 2019; 126(2):369–76.
19. Pugh GW, Hughes DE. Inhibition of autoagglutination of Moraxella bovis by 10% magnesium chloride. Appl Microbiol 1970;19(1):201–3.
20. Gard J, Taylor D, Maloney R, et al. Preliminary evaluation of hypochlorous acid spray for treatment of experimentally induced infectious bovine keratoconjunctivitis. Bovine Pract 2016;50(2):180–9.

Moving?

Make sure your subscription moves with you!

To notify us of your new address, find your **Clinics Account Number** (located on your mailing label above your name), and contact customer service at:

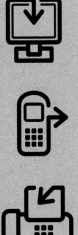

Email: **journalscustomerservice-usa@elsevier.com**

800-654-2452 (subscribers in the U.S. & Canada)
314-447-8871 (subscribers outside of the U.S. & Canada)

Fax number: 314-447-8029

Elsevier Health Sciences Division
Subscription Customer Service
3251 Riverport Lane
Maryland Heights, MO 63043

*To ensure uninterrupted delivery of your subscription, please notify us at least 4 weeks in advance of move.

ELSEVIER

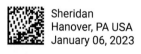